BALANCED MIND BALANCED LIFE

BALANCED MIND BALANCED LIFE

Adult colouring book combined with mindfulness art therapy and more!

Joe Aguilus

Saklolo

Australia

2024

Copyright 2024 Joe Aguilus

First Published in Australia in 2024 by *Saklolo*

889 / 585 Little Collins Street, Melbourne VIC 3000 Australia

ISBN: 978-1-7637724-0-3

All Rights Reserved. No part of this work can be transmitted or reproduced in any form including print, electronic, photocopying, scanning, mechanical, or recording without prior written permission from the author.

The contents of this book reflect the author's personal views and research. This book is not meant to be used, nor should it be used, to diagnose or treat any medical condition, including any diagnosed or undiagnosed mental health condition. The book is in no way intended to suggest any cure or treatment for any mental health condition or any other medical condition of any kind. For any diagnosis or treatment of any medical issue, we strongly advise that readers consult their own doctor or physician, psychologist, or counsellor as most appropriate. Neither the author nor the publisher is responsible for any medical or health needs from which the reader, or any person they know, may suffer. They are not liable for any damages or negative consequences for any treatment, action, application, or preparation used by any person, or their associates, who read this book. Advice and conclusions herein are drawn from standard and readily available research and articles and evidence sourced as referenced.

This book is published and sold with the understanding that neither the publisher nor the author is either engaged, or qualified, to offer any type of medical advice. Neither the author nor the publisher shall be liable for any physical, psychological, emotional, financial, commercial, or other damages, loss or other unwanted consequences of any kind. Our views and rights are the same: the reader and their associates are responsible for their own choices, actions, and consequences.

Dedication

To the readers who have taken the courageous step to recognize the importance of their mental health, I extend my heartfelt gratitude. Your willingness to acknowledge the areas in which you can grow and improve is a testament to your strength and resilience. The journey toward better well-being often begins with a single, challenging step, and I commend you for engaging in this transformative process. May you find inspiration, hope, and healing as you navigate your path toward a brighter, more fulfilling life.

Contents

About the Author ix

Preface xi

Introduction 1

Chapter 1   A Disease of our Age? A summary of how to help our mental health. 3

Chapter 2   Eating and Drinking for Mental Health – A tasty way to stay in shape 9

Chapter 3   Exercise – Good for the heart; great for the brain 21

Chapter 4   Sleep, Brain Work and Art – Balm for the Mind 26

Chapter 5   Mates, Mindfulness and Maintaining Balance 36

Chapter 6   Summing it All Up 44

Chapter 7   The Art of Now: Colouring Your Way to Mindfulness 47

Chapter 8   ❦ Comprehensive Daily Wellness & Growth Template 247

Bibliography: 251

Useful Resources 255

About the Author

Joe Aguilus is a man shaped by experience, a voice of empathy, and an advocate who understands the intricacies of mental health. His journey began as an immigrant from the Philippines, where he set foot in Australia over two decades ago. From those humble beginnings, Joe built a life, navigating the challenges of both personal and professional worlds. His career began with international airlines, a path that exposed him to the complexities of human interaction, culture, and growth. These early experiences planted the seeds of resilience, adaptability, and an understanding of the human condition that would later bloom into his writing and advocacy.

As Joe ventured further into his professional life, his interests expanded. He gained expertise in migration law, which allowed him to help others facing the uncertainties of relocation and cultural adaptation. This legal knowledge, combined with his work as a small business owner, content creator, and community advocate, gave him a multi-dimensional view of the world. It also deepened his sense of empathy. Joe's involvement in Human Resources, specifically in learning and development, honed his ability to foster growth and resilience within organizations—a skill he seamlessly weaves into his writing about mental well-being.

But it's not just his professional life that has shaped him; Joe's personal experiences have also fuelled his passion. As he pursued legal training, he discovered the powerful intersection between justice, mental health, and personal transformation. The law became another avenue through which he could advocate for others, aiming to ensure that people, especially those in vulnerable situations, have their voices heard. This understanding of fairness, combined with his own transformative journey, makes Joe's writing not only informative but deeply personal.

Joe's approach to mental health is both practical and heartfelt. He draws from his vast experience in change management, offering readers the tools they need to make positive changes in their own lives. His book doesn't just scratch the surface—it dives deep, addressing the often-unseen emotional struggles people face. With authenticity and compassion, Joe provides a guiding light for those navigating the complexities of mental health, offering strategies and insights that are grounded in both professional knowledge and personal understanding.

In the pages of his book, Joe's voice resonates with readers. He is not just an author, but a companion on the journey toward personal growth and resilience. His words inspire, providing practical guidance that readers can apply to their own lives. Joe's writing stands out because it combines the rigor of his background in Human Resources and legal studies with the warmth of someone who has walked the path of transformation himself. He reminds his readers that they are not alone and that through empathy, resilience, and self-discovery, they can find their own way forward.

Joe's work is more than a book—it is a beacon of hope. It empowers individuals to embrace their own mental well-being, helping them find strength in their challenges. His dedication to promoting strong mental health is a testament to his belief in a more compassionate society, where justice and empathy walk hand in hand. Through his writing, Joe leaves a lasting mark, encouraging his readers to develop their own resilience and to never stop growing. It's this commitment to change, to well-being, and to justice that makes Joe a writer who not only understands mental health but lives and breathes it in everything he does.

Preface

More than twenty years ago, I set foot in Australia with only hope and ambition, not knowing the profound transformations and challenges that would shape my path. Looking back now, this book reflects the lessons and insights born from both personal struggles and professional growth. My hope is that these reflections will inspire you to walk your own path with resilience, balance, and compassion.

Across my career—from international airlines to migration law, from small business ownership to corporate development—I've witnessed the vital role of mental well-being in leading a fulfilling life. True well-being reaches beyond simply managing stress or practicing mindfulness; it's about nurturing harmony among mind, body, and spirit. Within these pages, I share practical strategies drawn from my experiences and from evidence-based practices, whether to support your own well-being or to help others on their journey.

This book wouldn't be complete without acknowledging the hurdles I faced while advocating for fair and safe practices. When I raised concerns about repeated unsafe practices within Australia's Department of Home Affairs, I faced two significant privacy breaches. The first privacy breach, in 2021, came soon after my initial complaint, disrupting my business, damaging client trust, and devastating my new skincare startup.

Hoping for fair resolution, I entered a conciliation process organized by the Office of the Australian Information Commissioner (OAIC) with genuine faith in the process. However, instead of resolution, I found myself confronting intensified intimidation tactics from the Department, with a cadre of lawyers pressuring me throughout the conciliation in July 2022. It was deeply unsettling to learn that the OAIC—an agency meant to provide oversight—had failed to inform me about such aggressive tactics. Following this experience, a second privacy breach soon after the July 2022 conciliation session left me feeling silenced and pressured into submission, compounded by an offensive and unwarranted letter from their lawyers

Seeking accountability, I reached out to multiple government agencies, including Victoria Police, the Australian Federal Police, the Commonwealth Ombudsman, the newly established National Anti-Corruption Commission, and even the Prime Minister's office. Yet, none took steps to address these repeated offenses by public officials, which inflicted significant harm on my practice and well-being. Despite providing the OAIC with substantial evidence of these violations and their severe impact on my health, career, and finances, the agency ultimately chose not to investigate, dismissing my case as 'not complex' in November 2024.

These experiences taught me that true resilience lies in finding ways to stay cantered in the face of relentless challenges. They underscored the importance of self-care, self-advocacy, and safeguarding one's mental well-being in a world that isn't always fair. I share this story here because I believe deeply in the power of balance, even in times of adversity.

What makes this book unique is its holistic perspective. Together, we'll explore how foundational elements like diet, exercise, and sleep impact mental health, the healing power of creative outlets, and how simple activities—like the included colouring exercises—can release and process emotions. We'll discuss the value of social connections, self-reflection, and the courage to seek professional support. Each chapter draws on my background in Human Resources, learning and development, and my experiences as an immigrant adapting to new environments.

This book is not about quick fixes; it's a guide for meaningful change, with practical tools to nurture your mental well-being. Whether you're aiming to build resilience, deepen relationships, or gain insight into life's complexities, these tools are here to meet you where you are, offering a steady compass for your journey.

Remember, prioritizing your mental well-being is an act of strength. Life's challenges are as varied as we are, and this book honours that diversity with adaptable strategies suited to your unique needs. As you embrace these exercises and the art of self-care, know that this book is more than words—it's a companion in your pursuit of balance and fulfillment.

With empathy and hope

Joe Aguilus, MBA, MBus (IRHRM)
BSc (Tourism), GCertAusMigrationLawPrac
Melbourne, Australia
November 2024

Introduction

'Don't judge each day by the harvest that you reap but by the seeds that you plant'
Robert Stevenson[1]

In today's world, mental health issues are finally receiving the recognition they deserve, breaking free from centuries of silence and stigma. Over generations, our societies instilled in us the belief that mental health problems were something to be hidden away, shrouded in shame, often leading to misunderstanding and isolation. But times are changing. We're confronting a global challenge, one that affects us all. Prominent figures like Miley Cyrus, Prince Harry – who faced the heart-wrenching loss of his mother as a young child at boarding school – and swimmer Ian Thorpe have bravely shared their personal battles with mental health. This marks a significant turning point, even in the world of sports, especially male-dominated sports. Notable athletes like cricketer Marcus Trescothick and footballer Dele Alli are now openly discussing their own experiences. Finally, the age-old pressure to keep mental health issues concealed is fading.

The moment for change has arrived. Mental health disorders can be as corrosive as the most severe physical illnesses. At their worst, they can lead to the same tragic outcomes as the most severe forms of cancer, ischemia, or any other terminal condition. They subtly creep into every corner of our lives, often perpetuating themselves in relentless cycles: poor sleep can lead to mental health problems, which, in turn, make it harder to sleep well. These conditions, long shrouded in secrecy, thrive within the most destructive cycles of human existence.

But we are not powerless. We can take charge of our mental well-being, not just to improve it, but to maintain it at a consistently high level. This book is here to provide practical suggestions for achieving that. We'll explore various aspects of our lifestyle, from the food we eat to the exercise we engage in, and even the ways we keep our brain active. We'll also explore the crucial benefits of social interaction and tackle the deceptively simple yet profoundly challenging task of maintaining a positive outlook, with all the profound benefits it can bring. This book will guide us towards greater self-awareness, making it easier to recognize when we have concerns that require our attention.

---

[1] 'Robert Louis Stevenson', Robert Louis Stevenson Quotes (Web Page) <https://www.brainyquote.com/quotes/robert_louis_stevenson_101230>.

One important note – this book does not focus on high-level mental illnesses like schizophrenia or bipolar disorder. Those conditions remain the domain of highly qualified clinicians – individuals who have undergone years of rigorous training and are experts in their field. Instead, this book is all about practical ways to enhance our lifestyle, with the hope of enabling us to build a more honest and forward-thinking perspective on our emotional state. This, in turn, will help us address and prevent both short and long-term concerns about our mental well-being.

In the journey of life, we all inevitably encounter moments of fear, frustration, and times when we feel overwhelmed. These are just a few of the negative emotions that touch our lives from time to time. They are inherent to our human experience and often serve as signals, prompting important changes. To navigate these inevitable challenges effectively, it's crucial to first recognise them and then address them in positive ways. Implementing these strategies takes time and consistency; they cannot be mastered overnight. Through active practice and the application of the lessons we'll learn, we can gradually nurture a sense of happiness and fulfilment in our lives.

So, it's crucial to assess our habits and determine whether they are benefiting or hindering us. Where we find the latter, we need to be open to making necessary changes to reverse our decline and embark on a journey toward thriving.

This book aims to be our friendly guide on that journey. It's a resource that combines a professional understanding of mental health with a compassionate and approachable tone. Our goal is to provide the readers with the tools and insights needed to enhance their mental well-being, in a way that feels achievable and sustainable for their everyday life.

As we embark on this journey towards better mental health, we need to keep in mind that it's not just about addressing problems when they arise; it's about building a strong foundation for lifelong well-being. By embracing the practical suggestions and insights offered in this book, we're taking proactive steps to enhance our emotional and mental health. Whether we're looking to overcome temporary challenges or seeking to maintain long-term well-being, the principles and guidance shared here can be our compass.

This book is our partner in creating a more resilient, positive, and fulfilling mental journey. Remember, we're not alone in this process. Together, let's embark on a path toward greater mental well-being, one that empowers us to thrive, no matter the challenges that life may bring.

A Disease of our Age? A summary of how to help our mental health.

'It is health that is the real wealth and not pieces of gold and silver'
Mahatma Gandhi[2]

In the intricate blend of modern existence, mental health has emerged as a key aspect, influencing the lives of millions of people across the globe. The relentless pace of contemporary life, coupled with multifaceted stressors, has propelled mental health to the forefront of public consciousness. This comprehensive exploration seeks to untangle the complexities surrounding mental well-being, investigate into the interplay of diet, exercise, and stress, and provide a roadmap for fostering resilience and vitality in the face of life's challenges.

I. Understanding the Landscape

A. Global Perspectives on Mental Health

The prevalence of mental health issues is a global concern, going beyond borders and cultures. In Australia, one in five individuals acknowledges a mental health illness,[3] a figure that mirrors the challenges faced by one in four Americans.[4] This phenomenon emphasizes the universal nature of mental health challenges and serves as a call to action for understanding and addressing the factors that contribute to this alarming trend.

B. Hidden Struggles: Unreported Mental Health Issues

While statistics provide a snapshot of reported cases, the iceberg illustration competently describes the hidden struggles beneath the surface. A substantial number of individuals grapple with mental health concerns silently, either due to societal stigma or a lack of awareness regarding the origin of their distress. Untangling the complexities surrounding mental health requires acknowledging the hidden struggles that contribute to the broader landscape of well-being.

---

[2]'Mahatma Gandhi', Mahatma Gandhi Quotes (Web Page) <https://www.brainyquote.com/quotes/mahatma_gandhi_109078>.
[3]'Australian Institute of Health and Welfare', Prevalence and impact of mental illness (Web Page) < https://www.aihw.gov.au/mental-health/overview/prevalence-and-impact-of-mental-illness>.
[4]'Johns Hopkins Medicine', Mental Health Disorder Statistics (Web Page) <https://www.hopkinsmedicine.org/health/wellness-and-prevention/mental-health-disorder-statistics>.

C. The Global Burden: United Nations' Perspective

A staggering figure from the United Nations reveals that approximately a billion people worldwide grapple with diagnosed mental health conditions.[5] This figure encompasses diverse nations,[6] including those where awareness and reporting mechanisms are still in their infancy.[7] The global burden of mental health issues requires a delicate understanding of the socio-cultural,[8] economic,[9] and environmental factors that contribute to this pervasive challenge.[10]

Based on this, the relentless tsunami of mental health challenges globally appears poised to persist, fuelled by a combination of factors exacerbating its prevalence. Firstly, an increasing awareness surrounding mental health issues has sparked more individuals to actively pursue diagnosis and treatment. Secondly, the relentless pressures of society, including economic instability, social isolation, and environmental strains, continue to chew away at mental well-being. Thirdly, demographic transitions, marked by aging populations and rapid urbanization, threaten to blend the complexities of mental health struggles. Encouragingly, there has been a gradual erosion of the stigma encircling mental health, inspiring sufferers to step forward and seek help. Nevertheless, collective efforts such as bolstering access to mental health services and dismantling societal taboos are crucial to strengthen the relentless advance of this crisis. In essence, while the exact trajectory may fluctuate across regions, grappling with the multifaceted roots of mental health, is the key to curbing its enduring impact.

II. Diet: The Foundation of Mental Well-being

A. The Mind-Body Connection

The age-old saying, 'We are what we eat', takes on new significance in the realm of mental health. The relationship between diet and mental well-being is complex and multifaceted.[11] Beyond the primitive understanding of fullness and hunger, our dietary choices impact mood, cognitive function, and overall mental resilience. Untangling the complexities of this connection requires a deep dive into the intersection of nutrition and mental health.

---

[5]'United Nations', Nearly one billion people have a mental disorder: WHO (Web Page) <https://news.un.org/en/story/2022/06/1120682>.
[6]Ibid.
[7]'United Nations', *Nearly one billion people have a mental disorder*: WHO (Web Page) <https://news.un.org/en/story/2022/06/1120682>.
[8]Ibid.
[9]Ibid.
[10]Ibid.
[11]'Mental Health Foundation', Diet and mental health (Web Page) <https://www.mentalhealth.org.uk/explore-mental-health/a-z-topics/diet-and-mental-health>.

B. Consistency in Eating: A Key Pillar

The modern, hectic lifestyle often undermines the importance of regular and nutritious eating. 'Hangry' episodes, a result of fluctuating blood sugar levels, serve as a tangible reminder of the immediate impact of irregular eating habits. This section explores the challenges posed by busy lives and emphasizes the significance of establishing a routine that prioritises consistent and healthy dietary habits.

C. Hydration: The Overlooked Component

While food sustains us, the importance of hydration in maintaining mental well-being cannot be overstated. Dehydration, akin to blood sugar lows, can induce a state of misery, influencing mood and cognitive function. Recognising the symbiotic relationship between proper fluid intake and mental resilience unveils a holistic approach to nurturing the mind.

D. Beyond Sustenance: The Impact of Specific Foods

While the importance of a varied, healthy diet is widely acknowledged, exploration into the specific impact of certain foods on mood and outlook adds a layer of sophistication to our dietary understanding. The upcoming chapters will meticulously explore how elements of our diet, from antioxidants to omega-3 fatty acids, play an important role in shaping our mental well-being.

III. Exercise: Cultivating Physical and Mental Resilience

A. The Holistic Benefits of Exercise

Physical fitness, intertwined with mental well-being, forms the crux of a resilient and vibrant existence. Aerobic exercises, ranging from vigorous activities like jogging and swimming to more accessible options like gardening and walking, contribute to enhanced blood circulation to the brain. This section provides a preliminary examination of how exercise positively influences the brain's ability to cope with stress and promotes overall mental resilience.

B. Integrating Exercise into Daily Life

In a world dominated by sedentary lifestyles, from desk jobs to TV binges and long gaming sessions, incorporating exercise into daily routines becomes essential for enhancing physical and mental well-being. Small adjustments, such as parking farther away or choosing stairs over elevators, accumulate into significant positive impacts on overall fitness. This chapter explores the practical aspects of seamlessly integrating exercise into our lives.

C. Neurological Impacts: Beyond Stress Management

The physiological impacts of aerobic exercise extend beyond stress management. This section explores into the intricate neurological mechanisms at play, emphasizing how increased blood flow positively affects the limbic system, which governs mood and motivation.[12] Understanding these neurological impacts lays the groundwork for a holistic approach to mental well-being through physical fitness.

IV. Stress: Decoding the Complex Framework

A. The Inevitability of Stress

Stress, an inherent component of the human experience, filter through every aspect of modern life. While it may be impossible to eradicate stress entirely, understanding its origins and manifestations is key to developing effective coping strategies. This section confronts the inevitability of stress and sets the stage for a thorough exploration of its diverse sources.

B. Physiological and Psychological Impact

The impact of stress, both on a physiological and psychological level, is profound. Studies from diverse disciplines showcase how severe stress can cause tangible damage to our bodies, rendering us more susceptible to diseases.[13] The physiological toll on the immune system,[14] and vital organs,[15] underscores the urgency of addressing stress as a silent adversary.

C. Identifying Sources: A Multifaceted Challenge

The multitude of stressors in modern life necessitates a refined understanding of their origins. Financial stresses, relationship challenges, historical traumas, emotional struggles, medical concerns, and political anxieties are among the various sources contributing to the complex landscape of stress. Breaking down this intricate web requires a personalized and comprehensive approach

---

[12]'Dementia Australia', How do our brains work? (Web Page) <https://www.dementia.org.au/news/how-do-our-brains-work>.
[13]Neil Schneiderman, Gail Ironson, and Scott D. Siege, 'Stress and health: Psychological, behavioural, and biological determinants' (2005) 1(1) *Annual Review of Clinical Psychology* 607.
[14]Tetsuya Mizokami et al, 'Stress and Thyroid Autoimmunity' (2004) 14(12) Thyroid 1047.
[15]K Brown-Grant, GW Harris and S Reichlin, 'The effect of emotional and physical stress on thyroid activity in the rabbit' (1954) 126(1) *The Journal of Physiology* 29.

V. Sources of Stress: A Deeper Dive

Navigating the Complexities of Stress: A Holistic Exploration

In the complex environment of human existence, stress weaves its threads through various dimensions, influencing our mental well-being. This in-depth exploration examines the diverse aspects of stress, examining its origins, manifestations, and potential strategies for resilience. By scrutinising financial stresses, relationship dynamics, historical echoes, emotional intricacies, medical challenges, and political influences, we aim to offer unique insights into navigating this complex terrain.

A. Financial Stresses:

The financial landscape is a profound source of stress, intertwining money concerns, career anxieties, job insecurities, and the delicate equilibrium of work-life balance. Beyond the surface, it significantly impacts mental health. In this section, we embark on a journey to unravel the intricate relationship between financial well-being and mental health. Strategies for navigating this complex terrain include financial literacy, prudent budgeting, and fostering a mindset that separates self-worth from monetary success.

B. Relationship Stresses:

Interpersonal dynamics wield considerable influence over mental well-being. Whether it's relationships with partners, children, parents, or friends, the difficulties of social connections contribute to the delicate balance of mental health. This segment examines into the complex interplay of relationships and stress, offering unique insights into fostering healthy connections. Communication, empathy, and setting boundaries emerge as key tools for mitigating the negative impact of relationships on mental well-being.

C. Historical Stresses:

The echoes of past traumas, failures, and losses reverberate through our present, shaping the contours of our mental well-being. A compassionate examination of individual narratives is essential to understanding the profound impact of historical stresses. This section calls for acknowledging the role of past experiences in shaping present mental health and advocates for therapeutic interventions to heal deep-seated wounds.

D. Emotional Stresses:

Emotions, ranging from natural anxiety to a sense of disappointment and fear of change, contribute additional layers to the complex terrain of stress. This segment explores into the detailed realm of emotional stresses, recognizing their significant influence on mental health. Strategies for emotional resilience include mindfulness practices, cultivating emotional intelligence, and seeking professional support to navigate the tumultuous waves of emotions.

E. Medical Stresses:

Health concerns, both personal and familial, along with broader issues like pandemics, pose substantial challenges to mental well-being. This section investigates the intricate relationship between medical stresses and mental health, highlighting the need for a holistic approach to well-being. Encouraging a balance between physical and mental health, fostering a supportive community, and seeking professional guidance are crucial aspects of coping with medical stresses.

F. Political Stresses:

The socio-political landscape, rife with concerns about climate change, political perspectives, war, crime, and injustice, contributes to a pervasive sense of unease. Navigating the impact of political stresses on mental health requires a sophisticated understanding of contemporary societal challenges. This section explores the complexities of political influences, emphasizing the importance of informed civic engagement, establishing boundaries in media consumption, and cultivating resilience in the face of societal uncertainties.

In the kaleidoscope of stress, each facet contributes to the overall composition of our mental well-being. By understanding the intricate relationships between financial, relationship, historical, emotional, medical, and political stresses, individuals can embark on a journey towards resilience and holistic well-being. Navigating this multifaceted terrain requires a combination of self-awareness, interpersonal skills, and a proactive approach to mental health. In this exploration, we strive to provide a roadmap for individuals seeking to, not only cope with stress, but to thrive in the face of life's challenges.

VI. Conclusion: A Roadmap to Resilience

Navigating the intricacies of mental well-being demands a holistic approach that considers the interplay of diet, exercise, and stress. Over the remaining chapters, we embark on a journey to explore practical and accessible ways to enhance mental health, prevent its deterioration, and leverage its positive influence on our lives. This comprehensive exploration serves as a roadmap to resilience, recognizing the pivotal role of diet as the starting point for our transformative journey toward a nourished and resilient mind.

Eating and Drinking for Mental Health – A tasty way to stay in shape

'The doctor of the future will no longer treat the human frame with drugs, but rather will cure and prevent disease with nutrition'
Thomas Edison[16]

Exposing the Global Impact of Depression and Mental Health

Felice Jacka, the Professor of Nutritional Psychiatry at Deakin University and Director of the Food and Mood Centre, highlights a startling global issue in that depression has been recognized as the primary cause of disability worldwide.[17] The impact of this condition is profound, affecting various aspects of a person's life. A recent study highlights that depression can detrimentally influence working memory, leading to implications for learning and productivity.[18] The cycle of reduced ability and achievement in the face of depression can exacerbate the condition.[19]

Adding to the gravity of the situation, data from 2019 revealed that 1 in every 8 people,[20] approximately 970 million individuals globally,[21] were living with a mental disorder,[22] with anxiety and depressive disorders being the most prevalent.[23] The year 2020 witnessed a significant surge in the number of people grappling with anxiety and depressive disorders,[24] attributed to the COVID-19 pandemic,[25] with a 26% increase in anxiety and a 28% increase in major depressive disorders within just one year.[26] Despite the existence of effective prevention and treatment options,[27] a considerable portion of individuals with mental disorders lacks access

---

[16]'Thomas A Edison', Thomas A. Edison Quotes (Web Page) <https://www.brainyquote.com/quotes/thomas_a_edison_1063850>.
[17]'Felice Jacka', The fascinating connection between diet and depression (Web Page) <https://this.deakin.edu.au/self-improvement/the-fascinating-connection-between-diet-and-depression>.
[18]Steven Nikolin et al, 'An investigation of working memory deficits in depression using the n-back task: A systematic review and meta-analysis' (2021) 284 Journal of Affective Disorders 1.
[19]Ibid.
[20]'World Health Organization', Mental disorders (Web Page) <https://www.who.int/news-room/fact-sheets/detail/mental-disorders>.
[21]Ibid.
[22]Ibid.
[23]Ibid.
[24]Ibid.
[25]Ibid.
[26]Ibid.
[27]Ibid.

to adequate care.[28] Additionally, stigma,[29] discrimination,[30] and human rights violations compound the challenges.[31]

Amidst these alarming statistics, Jacka emphasizes that one potent means of safeguarding against mental health issues is adopting a healthy diet.[32] However, it's crucial to note the varying figures reported by official bodies on the global prevalence of mental health illnesses, indicative of our ongoing efforts to comprehend the full extent of this pervasive issue. Nevertheless, there is a growing understanding of the pivotal role played by healthy and regular eating in bolstering emotional well-being.[33]

Junk Food's Impact: Highs to Lows in Mental Well-being

It often feels like a sinister plot – the universe conspiring with unhealthy food to lay a trap for us. Picture this: a classic Catch-22 scenario where our bodies, worn down and spirits sagging, crave a quick fix – a sugar or energy surge. And just at that vulnerable moment, like a cunning parasite, junk food emerges from the shadows, offering itself to our yearning bodies.

However, the satisfaction from this unholy alliance is short-lived. The initial energy rush bestowed by junk food is short-lived, leaving us in the clutches of a prolonged, energy-draining low. But the plot thickens. Alongside the transient burst of energy comes a barrage of harmful elements that we're all too familiar with – high salt and sugar content, digestive havoc, that uncomfortable bloated sensation, and a cocktail of highly processed, harmful additives and alien chemicals lying in wait to ambush our insides.

Even as junk food wreaks havoc, our bodies seem to conveniently forget the downsides, clinging onto the memory of that temporary high. So, when the blues strike again, our bodies, misguided by this selective amnesia, steer us back to the destructive embrace of snacks that masquerade as a solution.

The most direct link between junk food and the melancholy associated with a diet steeped in this modern opium is its impact on digestion. It's not just about the harmful content; it's the absence of essential nutrients crucial for a healthy mind and a thriving brain that inflicts the damage. The ripple effect on digestion unleashes a wave of unwanted mental health issues –

---

[28]'World Health Organization', Mental disorders (Web Page) <https://www.who.int/news-room/fact-sheets/detail/mental-disorders>.
[29]Ibid.
[30]Ibid.
[31]Ibid.
[32]'Felice Jacka', The fascinating connection between diet and depression (Web Page) <https://this.deakin.edu.au/self-improvement/the-fascinating-connection-between-diet-and-depression>.
[33]'BBC Food', How diet can affect your mental wellbeing (Web Page) < https://www.bbc.co.uk/food/articles/diet_wellbeing>.

think brain fog, that foggy inability to think clearly, and a persistent feeling of bloated sluggishness, just to name a couple of unwelcome side effects.

This detrimental journey doesn't stop there. Tied to these physical discomforts are companions like anxiety, mood swings, and a hair-trigger annoyance level – a less-than-ideal state for both us and those in our orbit. The realisation of this, only serves to deepen the emotional abyss.

What's the supposed solution? A burst of energy. And where does our loyal body direct us to seek it? The ever-enticing, ever-deceptive world of more junk food. The cycle perpetuates, and the plot thickens.

Junk Food's Seductive Trap: Unveiling Its Destructive Charm

Behold the malevolent maestro of culinary chaos – this dietary villain not only boasts a knack for tantalizing taste buds but also prides itself on swift availability. It's no mere coincidence that it's dubbed fast-food; it's a culinary sprinter with an agenda. While research extols the virtues of a wholesome, Mediterranean diet,[34] as the gold standard – the best, healthiest, and most sustainable – the reality is, who among us wants to embark on a culinary odyssey involving a cornucopia of fruits, nut-shelling escapades, or the gourmet preparation of fish when the siren call of a crisps-and-chocolate duo echoes from the cupboard?

Enter the seductive forces of salt and sweet – the dynamic duo that junk food masterfully wields to captivate our taste buds. Sometimes, in a feat of culinary alchemy, it manages to allure with both. It's a parasitic puppeteer, pulling the strings of our cravings with finesse, making us unwittingly fall in love with its destructive charm.

Now, a sporadic dalliance with junk food might not sound alarms, but for many, it fans the flames of an addictive yearning – a perilous inclination that extends beyond mere physical harm. The risks of a junk food-centric diet are not confined to the expanding waistline; they infiltrate the corridors of mental well-being, creating an unfortunate symbiosis. Loaded with an abundance of calories, junk food boldly contributes to our transformation into, well, let's say it plainly, chubbier versions of ourselves. The cunning part? Those calories take residence around our midriff, while the fats craftily settle in our arteries, orchestrating a symphony of slow and sluggish vibes. And as we sink into this physical torpor, the motivation to exercise becomes a distant memory, perpetuating a cycle of long-term physical harm and immediate mental health havoc.

---

[34]Marc Molendijk et al, 'Diet quality and depression risk: A systematic review and dose-response meta-analysis of prospective studies' (2018) 226 Journal of Affective Disorders 346.

So, if the quest is to banish or at least significantly diminish the presence of junk food from our diets, what culinary delights should grace our plates? Let's explore the path to a healthier, more nourishing feast.

Omega-3: Nourishing Mental Harmony and Joy

Enter the realm of nutritional wisdom, where the spotlight now shines brightly on the potent prowess of omega-3 fats – not merely guardians of mental well-being but virtuosos in enhancing it.[35] These elusive fats weave their magic in various delectable sources, a symphony of mental nourishment found in the depths of oily fish, like salmon, mackerel, sardines, and the quirky kippers. Nuts, with walnuts taking centre stage, and the unassuming seeds, especially the mighty chia, complete this nutritional ensemble.

Picture this: a sprinkle of chia seeds adorning your morning bowl of porridge, not just for a delightful crunch but as a mood-boosting prelude to your day. The intricate dance these omega-3 fats perform is nothing short of captivating. They navigate effortlessly through the intricate membrane of brain cells, engaging with molecules that hold the reins on our moods. Think of them as conductors orchestrating a symphony of emotional harmony within the brain.

But that's not all – these remarkable fats are more than mood maestros. They actively champion the cause of 'happy hormones' – dopamine and serotonin – coaxing their release by influencing nerve cell membranes in the brain. Picture it as a nutritional serenade for your well-being.

Wait, there's more. Omega-3 fats don a superhero cape with anti-inflammatory characteristics, emerging as champions in the battle against the ominous cloud of depression. In essence, they're not just nutrients; they're the unsung heroes that navigate the intricate pathways of our brain, promoting not just mental resilience but a symphony of joy within.

From Oily Fish to Granary Bread: The Art of Well-being on a Plate

Let's dive back into the delicious saga of nutrition, where the Mediterranean diet reigns supreme, a vibrant blend woven with fresh vegetables, an abundance of fruit, and a generous sprinkling of nuts and seeds. The gospel of health resonates through research findings,[36] declaring the remarkable power of this diet in reducing the looming threat of depression.[37] Red meats, cast as occasional guests, make fleeting appearances – once a week is plenty, and perhaps

---

[35]Jerome Sarris et al, 'Nutritional psychiatry: the present state of the evidence' (2020) 76(4) Proceedings of the Nutrition Society 427.
[36]Felice N Jacka et al, 'A randomised controlled trial of dietary improvement for adults with major depression (the 'SMILES' trial)' (2017) 15(1) BMC Medicine 1.
[37]Ibid.

even better every fortnight. In their stead, the spotlight turns to the ocean's bounty, with oily fish stealing the scene to provide us with the coveted omega-3 fats that fuel our thriving.

Now, notice the conspicuous absence of carbohydrates? Fear not, for they are not banished; they merely walk the path of enlightenment in their unprocessed, brown varieties. Brown rice, whole-wheat pastas, and the symphony of granary and whole grain breads take centre stage, transforming our plate into a canvas of health. Imagine a breakfast tableau – a bowl of slow-releasing energy in the form of porridge, adorned with succulent blueberries and seeds, perhaps sweetened to taste with a dollop of honey or slices of banana. It's not just breakfast; it's a symphony of health, a nourishing ode to physical and mental well-being.

And let's address the ever-present carb conundrum. The revelation that brown, whole-grain rice outshines its processed white counterpart or that a nutty, crunchy wholemeal loaf outperforms its sliced white counterpart should hardly come as a surprise. It's as basic, as basking in the nutritional sunlight we've been neglecting for far too long. And, when it comes to the bread debate, taste is the ultimate arbiter. Picture this: a thin slice of ham sandwiched between two pallid, dry-as-wit white slices versus a thick wedge of still-warm granary, crowned with crisp salad and a wedge of tangy cheddar. The choice is clear, not just for the palate but for the overall celebration of well-being.

A quick sidebar – dairy, often relegated to the shadows for its perceived fat content and allergy risks, gets a nod. While not hailed as a champion in enhancing mental well-being, moderation is the key unless you harbour specific allergies. So, let's savour the symphony of flavours, embracing the wisdom that a wholesome diet, not only fuels our bodies, but becomes a melody of joy for our minds.

Nourishing Minds: The Art and Science of Food Choices

Anyway, in the theatre of our supermarket choices, the star that often graces our basket is the sliced white bread, and our rice, steadfastly accompanying the mildly piquant Korma, tends to be of the stodgy white variety. Even our diligently boiled spaghetti emerges from its hot bath looking pale and pasty. Why, you ask? The answer, my friends, is a trio of factors entangled in a dance of psychology, science, and sheer convenience.

In the enigmatic realm of taste, it's surprising to learn that our taste buds aren't the sole architects of flavour perception. Instead, the first encounter with food is a visual affair. Our eyes send signals to the brain, laying the foundation for what to expect. The brain, ever the trusting companion, clings to this initial impression, despite contrary information from other senses. Behold the power of colour psychology – an orange drink is assumed to taste of oranges, a cake with a yellow drizzle is deemed lemony, but alas, brown pasta? It's associated with less palatable things – mud, dirt, bodily functions. Our brain, ever vigilant, sends out a warning of impending unpleasantness. Natural whole meal foods find themselves at a disadvantage before the taste buds even get a chance. Crafty manufacturers are privy to this game and employ the art of colour manipulation, enhancing their creations with enticing hues. A pudding with a hint of rotten eggs? No problem, drown it in yellow colouring and additives, and suddenly it's a delightful lemony treat, egg aftertaste be damned. It's a blend of psychology and science, perhaps oversimplified but undeniably clear in its message.

Convenience, that ever-enticing siren, enters the stage. Consider a freshly baked wholemeal loaf – perfect for lunch, an ideal complement to an evening salad, and suitable for morning toast. The birds might even join the feast on the third day. Now, contrast this with a highly processed white loaf – an instant sandwich supply for the week. Convenience often tilts the scales.

Identifying a diet that champions mental well-being isn't rocket science. It's a colourful canvas of variety, abundant fresh fruits and vegetables, a sprinkling of nuts and seeds, the bounty of fish, moderated carbs, and a generous serving of healthy proteins that won't clog our arteries with unwanted fats. Processed, convenience foods take a backseat in this harmonious ensemble, allowing the natural symphony of nutrition to take centre stage.

Social Feasts: A Recipe for Mental Well-being

Ah, the perpetual struggle in our hustle-filled lives – the elusive quest for time and motivation to craft wholesome meals. Yet, there's a beacon of hope that shines brighter when we dine in the company of others. There's an innate pleasure in conjuring up culinary delights for family, a partner, or friends. (By the way, having a partner can be a mental health booster[38]—like having a partner in crime against mental illness, if you will).

Now, for the solo dwellers among us, fear not; there's a remedy – make a social feast a weekly rendezvous, or better yet, a frequent one. Summon folks over and watch as the motivation to whip up a nutritious masterpiece skyrockets.

And let's address the ever-elusive time constraint. If we're candid with ourselves, time shouldn't be the hurdle it's made out to be. Why do we toil away at work? For most, it's to fund a life that we enjoy. But here's the reality check – how much enjoyment are we deriving if mental health concerns cast a shadow? Prioritise, my friend. Take a step back from the rat race, reassess, and

---

[38] Rodrigo J Carcedo et al, 'Association between sexual satisfaction and depression and anxiety in adolescents and young adults' (2020) 17(3) International journal of environmental research and public health 1.

suddenly, mental (and physical) health catapults to the summit of our life improvement wishlist. Those extra hours to impress the boss? Maybe not worth it.

Now, let's pivot to the solitary dining dilemma. Does the prospect of spending an hour crafting a delectable dinner enthral us when it's devoured in five minutes? Especially when we're hunched in front of the TV, barely savouring the fruits of our culinary labour. It's tempting to opt for the microwave's swift embrace and bang out a processed meal with far less fuss.

In the grand story of life, the act of eating socially emerges as a powerful catalyst, not just for the joy of shared meals, but as a motivator for prioritizing our mental and physical well-being. So, let's break bread together, relish the communal joy, and reclaim our time for the things that truly enrich our lives.

Culinary Delights: Fresh to Frozen

Let's dive into the realm of culinary wisdom, armed with tips that might sound like the sage advice of our grandmas – and trust me, grandmas are the unsung heroes of common sense. So, buckle up for some kitchen revelations that can turn our hurried Sunday lunch dash into a more mindful and satisfying experience.

Now, while we all know that fresh fruits and veggies are the rock stars of nutrition, let's not underestimate their frozen, or tinned counterparts. They're like, the unsung heroes – almost as good, require minimal prep, and the bonus? The saucepan practically cleans itself as it simmers away, transforming mundane tasks into a culinary delight.

Ah, the dreaded post-meal cleanup – a thundercloud over our Wagga, as if the universe conspired against our solo dining escapades. But fear not, turn the tables by doing the dishes as you go. Sure, the total time in the soapsuds might not differ much, but the mental boost of knowing your only post-meal chore is popping the plate in the dishwasher is a game-changer. And let's face it, finding ways to uplift our mental well-being is the heart of this culinary adventure.

Planning is the unsung hero here. Instead of grappling with dinner fatigue at the end of a long day, channel your inner chef on a buzzing Sunday afternoon. With the radio playing your jam, whip up a storm using the carefully chosen ingredients from your weekly shop. Whether it's a tangy, flavourful vegetable lasagna (wholemeal pasta, obviously) for a party of eight or just one, the process remains the same. Prepare, cook, slice, and freeze. You've got a portion in the fridge for later, one for tonight, and six in the freezer for the weeks ahead. Box up some salads for the next few days; they'll keep. The salmon you whip up? It's good for up to three days if stored properly! Suddenly, your freezer is a treasure trove of healthy, ready-to-go meals. No bloated feelings, no processed food aftermath. Just pure satisfaction, a happy gut, and a calorie count that won't tip the scales. It's a virtuous circle – a mental equilibrium that not only maintains but perpetuates itself. We feel happy, and that happiness bring about even more joy. Cheers to the culinary wisdom that nourishes both body and mind!

Supplements: Mental Health Sidekicks

Time to unravel the nutritional secrets that play a harmonious tune with our mental well-being. A symphony of vitamins takes the stage, each with its unique role in the grand performance of our mental health. Picture this: the spotlight shines on the vital trio of vitamin A, C, and the virtuoso B, with B12 leading the orchestration. Then, there's the sunshine maestro, vitamin D, the mystical zinc, the calming magnesium, and the enchanting folate. It's like assembling the Avengers for our mental resilience.

Here's the plot twist – when we're deficient in these nutritional superheroes, the spectre of depression and its disorderly companions looms larger.[39] But fear not, for the culinary superheroes are here to save the day. Healthy foods, the unsung carriers of these essential vitamins, stand ready to be our nutritional guardians.

Yet, the plot thickens – enter supplements, the trusty sidekicks. When the spotlight shifts, and we find ourselves in need of a vitamin top-up, supplements swoop in like caped crusaders, ensuring we get the nutrients where and when we need them. It's like having a nutritional backup plan, a convenient and efficient way to ensure our mental fortress remains fortified.

So, whether it's savouring a plate of vitamin-packed goodness or unleashing the power of supplements, our nutritional arsenal stands ready to champion mental well-being. It's a tale of vitamins, superheroes, and a resilient mind – the blockbuster we've all been waiting for!

---

[39]T S Sathyanarayana Rao et al, 'Understanding nutrition, depression and mental illnesses' (2008) 50(2) Indian Journal of Psychiatry 77.

Sip Smart: Navigating Hydration for Mental Well-being

Let's embark on the delightful journey of sustenance and hydration, where eating and drinking – in the grandest sense – become the companions of our mental well-being. Picture this: the elixir of life, water, takes centre stage. If the pure simplicity of water doesn't tickle your taste buds, fear not. Enter the sparkling varieties or elevate your hydration game with a splash of lime or lemon. Pro tip: keep a bottle in the freezer for a day-long frosty embrace. Icy water, for many, is a refreshing oasis compared to its tepid counterpart.

Now, onto the nectar that fuels many of our daily adventures – coffee. Despite the (admittedly reasonable) caffeine cautions, a cup or two a day emerges as a hero, delivering a repertoire of health benefits.[40] But here's the plot twist – caffeine is a sleep saboteur. So, let's cap our coffee consumption before the clock strikes afternoon and certainly bid it farewell after dinner.

Beverages often have a sneaky diuretic impact, playing hide-and-seek with our hydration goals. Yet, fear not, for a cup of tea steps in as a hydration ally. And for those craving a fruity symphony, half a glass of juice becomes the pleasant gateway to the benefits of fruits and vegetables. A word of caution – mind the sugar content in packaged juices. The wise investment? A juicer. It not only ensures your orange juice is free of additives but also doubles as a money-saving maestro in the long run.

In this culinary and liquid fusion, hydration becomes an art, and our choices a symphony of well-being. So, here's to sipping wisely, embracing the icy refreshment, and relishing the subtle notes of health in every drop. Cheers to the liquid poetry that nourishes both body and mind!

Beyond the Glass: Unveiling the Risks of Alcohol and the Shadows of Food Addiction

Ah, the great alcohol debate – a quagmire of conflicting evidence that could make your head spin faster than a carousel. But let's tiptoe through this minefield with caution, acknowledging that too much of the spirited elixir isn't exactly a recipe for mental health success. An occasional glass of red or bubbles (or your drink of choice), on the other hand, might just be a harmless relaxation, especially if it's entwined with the delightful dance of social interaction. It's like a delicate balance, where the benefits of a social toast perhaps outweigh the potential pitfalls of the alcohol itself, at least, in terms of our mental well-being.

---

[40]'Kimberly Holland', How many cups of coffee a day are safe? (Web Page) < https://www.healthline.com/health-news/6-cups-of-coffee-a-day-is-safe-but-more-isnt-healthy>.

Yet, tread carefully, for the real trouble brews when alcohol becomes the masquerade for our mental struggles. Picture it as a treacherous journey on a winding road, and your vehicle? A car with dodgy brakes heading straight for a cliff edge. Not exactly a scenic route to mental serenity.

Now, let's shift gears to the lesser-known territory of food addiction, a formidable force that lurks in the shadows. It's not just about craving a snack when you're not particularly hungry,[41] it's an addiction that echoes the same ominous health concerns, as its notorious counterparts – alcohol or drug addiction, be it prescription or illicit. Picture it as a dark dance with mental well-being, each step leading us further into the abyss.

And here's the twist – addiction, whether to alcohol, substances, or food, isn't a puzzle you can solve by flipping through the pages of a book. It's a labyrinth that demands external, professional guidance. Seeking help is the compass that can navigate this intricate maze, steering us away from the cliffs and guiding us towards the brighter, healthier horizons of mental well-being. It's a journey worth taking, with the right support steering the wheel.

Savouring Symphonies: A Digestive Dance in Nutritional Grace

It's not just about the when and what of our culinary escapades, but also the sacred how. Picture this: perched upright, engaging in a culinary tango with a tangy-dressed salad and a side of (brown) rice. This isn't just about proper posture; it's a digestion dance party. By sitting tall, we're giving the green light for the nutrients to waltz through our system, doing the tango of nourishment. Now, contrast this with the cozy slouch on the sofa, tray precariously perched on the lap, Netflix playing the leading role. Sure, it's a comfort haven, but the aftermath includes the fiery turmoil of acid reflux, and worse, a squandered nutritional feast. The relaxation might feel sweet, but the price? Not so much.

Now, let's pivot to the communal symphony of social eating. Sharing a meal isn't just a leisurely affair; it's a rhythmic slowdown in our typical culinary sprint. We're all guilty of inhaling our food too swiftly. But when we trade our solo dining sprint for a leisurely stroll, the benefits are manifold. It's not just about unwinding; it's about the emotional rendezvous of connecting with family or enriching the bond of friendship.

So, let's savour our meals in the upright posture of nutritional grace, allowing the flavours to mingle with our senses. And when the occasion calls for communal feasting, let's linger a little longer, relishing the flavours, the camaraderie, and the sheer joy of shared culinary tales. It's not just eating; it's a symphony of experiences, where the how transforms the act into a masterpiece.

---

[41]'Kris Gunnars', How to overcome food addiction (Web Page) < https://www.healthline.com/nutrition/how-to-overcome-food-addiction>.

Microbiome Symphony: Unveiling the Gut-Brain Tango

Decoding the mysteries of the intricate tango between our gut and brain is a journey of continuous discovery. In the latest chapter of this saga, a report emerged, shining a spotlight on the microbiome—the bustling ecosystem where micro-organisms set up shop in our gut.[42] It's not just a backstage feature; it's the director, influencing brain function,[43] orchestrating behaviour, and conducting a symphony that reverberates through the corridors of mental health.[44] Yet, as we eagerly sip from the fountain of understanding, a word of caution emerges. The rapid pace of our insights is both a gift and a riddle. Yes, indulging in a diet that flirts with the boundaries of healthy is undoubtedly a boon. The impact on our mental well-being is palpable, a dance of nourishment. However, the intricate details of this relationship remain a puzzle, a canvas still unfurling with nuances waiting to be discovered. It's like reading a captivating novel with each turn of the page revealing a new layer of the plot. The journey to unravel the depth of this connection is as tantalizing as the flavours of a well-prepared dish, and the adventure has only just begun.

Sip, Bite, Socialize: Crafting Your Anthem for a Healthier Life

Let's distil the essence from this chapter: the rhythmic cadence of eating and staying hydrated regularly is our secret anthem. Picture this: a harmonious melody of a healthy, well-rounded diet, adorned with the sweet notes of omega-3-rich foods. And, as a weekly rendezvous, sprinkle in a social feast or two. It's not a culinary revolution; it's a subtle culinary symphony, orchestrating emotional crescendos in our lives. These tweaks to our culinary routine won't unleash chaos; instead, they might unfurl emotionally significant moments. That, in itself, is reason enough to dip our toes into the pool of healthy eating. So, let's embark on this culinary adventure, where the flavours of well-being await, promising not disruption but a gentle dance of positive change. Cheers to the delightful notes of a healthier, happier life!

Conclusion:

In a nutshell, the narrative underscores the vital connection between what we eat and our mental well-being. Depression's impact on cognition and the disruptive influence of junk food highlights the urgent need for a nourishing diet as a robust defence against mental health disorders. Choosing for a Mediterranean diet, rich in omega-3 foods, emerges as a positive

---

[42] Anastasia I Petra et al, 'Gut-microbiota-brain axis and its effect on neuropsychiatric disorders with suspected immune dysregulation' (2022) 44(1) Clinical Therapeutics 10.
[43] Ibid.
[44] Ibid.

alternative. Practical strategies like culinary wisdom, planning, and communal dining offer solutions to time constraints. The symphony of vitamins, hydration, and balanced alcohol consumption reinforces the role of food in nurturing mental resilience, while the gut-brain connection adds an intricate layer. In essence, this culinary journey promises a gentle dance of positive change for a healthier, happier life. Cheers to the delightful notes of well-being!

Exercise – Good for the heart; great for the brain

'Australia is an outdoor country. People only go inside to use the toilet.
And that's only a recent development'
Barry Humphries[45]

In the exploration that lies ahead, we shall embark on a quest to unravel the mysteries surrounding exercise and its profound impact on mental health. Three key questions shall guide us through this enlightening journey: What form of exercise best supports mental well-being? What specific advantages does this chosen exercise confer upon our mental health? Lastly, how can we seamlessly incorporate and sustain this exercise routine in our lives? The landscape of fitness enthusiasts can be divided into various camps, each stationed at different altitudes on the metaphorical exercise Everest.

At the pinnacle of this Everest stand those who engage in regular, strenuous workouts. Just below, at the cusp of the final ascent, are individuals who recognize the importance of exercise but approach it with a tinge of reluctance. Nestled in the base camp are those content with occasional walks, their exercise endeavours limited to these casual strolls. Lastly, there exists a group for whom a sporadic Google search about the grand mountain, is sufficient to satiate their curiosity.

For those navigating the upper echelons of fitness, the path to improving mental health might seem well-trodden. However, even dedicated exercisers are not immune to mental health challenges. The very dedication that drives them to exercise rigorously may lead to pitfalls such as obsessive behaviour, over-competitiveness, and a constant need for self-esteem boosts. Additionally, the risk of injuries, like muscle strains, can potentially impede the very activity that fulfils their need for exercise. Despite reaching this chapter, recognizing that their exercise routine could contribute more to overall mental well-being is a significant step.

Yet, for this group, a chasm often exists between knowing what should be done and finding the motivation to act on this knowledge. Even once initiated, maintaining the requisite level of exercise to sustain and enhance mental health can pose a formidable challenge. Exercise is akin to gardening, a notion we'll dig into later as a form of informal exercise. Some find joy in maintaining to flower beds and trimming hedges, relishing both the process and the results achieved. Others view the impending lawn mowing as a burdensome task, compounded by the

---

[45]'Barry Humphries', 50+ Ripper Australian quotes, slang and sayings (Web Page) < https://aussietourist.com.au/australian-quotes-instagram-captions/>.

knowledge that the neatness attained is ephemeral. A subset of this group may even relinquish control, allowing the garden to run wild, making the reclamation of overgrown foliage an even more arduous task.

Metaphors aside, the opening chapter underscored the efficacy of aerobic exercise in addressing mental health issues and promoting overall well-being. However, it's crucial not to become overly fixated on the scientific intricacies supporting this conclusion. At its core, exercise, in any form, is beneficial for us. Yet, a psychological hurdle emerges when exercise transforms into a 'must-do' task, akin to the obligatory ingestion of cod liver oil or tackling a weighty Victorian classic. When viewed as a chore, akin to bathroom cleaning, the likelihood of evasion increases.

Many can relate to the mental gymnastics involved in convincing ourselves to forgo exercise—whether it's because it's a Sunday or due to the exertions of the previous day. Granted, not everyone shares this sentiment; there are those who genuinely relish exercise. To the exercise enthusiasts, this chapter extends its appreciation, but it's not the focus of our exploration.

The silver lining lies in the fact that we need not embark on Herculean efforts to reap the rewards of exercise. The very notion of 'work' associated with exercise can be reframed as 'pleasure,' 'movement,' 'taking the air,' or simply 'fun'. Language matters; let us adopt a lexicon that transforms exercise into a positive pursuit rather than a tedious chore. The revelation is that we don't require excessive amounts of exercise to unlock its benefits. A mere 150 minutes or two and a half hours per week,[46] as long as it elevates our heart rate even slightly, sets in motion a cascade of benefits.

The key to integrating exercise seamlessly into our daily lives lies in discovering the method that resonates with us. It need not be intricate or financially burdensome. The beauty of exercise lies in its perpetuity—it keeps on giving. By enhancing mental health, it elevates our mood and boosts self-esteem, transforming us from a disgruntled individual to a beacon of happiness. Consequently, it doesn't coerce us into action but rather breeds a genuine desire to partake. The only challenge lies in taking that initial step.

Honesty, as they say, is the best policy. If we find physical exercise to be a bit of a drag, we need to work on shifting our mindset. The good news is that with the right approach, the effort required to find reward doesn't have to be overwhelming. Our goal is to make exercise emotionally accessible, transforming it from a burdensome task, into something we genuinely enjoy.

---

[46]'Mental Health Foundation', How to look after your mental health using exercise (Web Page) < https://www.mentalhealth.org.uk/explore-mental-health/publications/how-look-after-your-mental-health-using-exercise>.

One: The New Year's Day Approach – Join a Gym

Consider the New Year's Day Approach—join a gym. Here, the emphasis isn't on sculpting a six-pack (unless that's your aspiration) but on getting your heart pumping. Three ten-minute sessions a day, five times a week, can achieve the desired results. Spice things up by diversifying the equipment you use to keep things interesting.

Two: The Invigorating Approach – Go for a Swim

For those who find joy in the water, consider swimming. Beyond being a comprehensive physical workout, it engages a variety of muscles and offers substantial mental health benefits. If the monotony of pool laps doesn't appeal, venture into open water or wild swimming. Joining a club ensures safety, as these activities are more enjoyable and safer when done in a group setting.

Three: The Enlightening Approach – Take Up a New Hobby

Explore the enlightening approach—adopt a new hobby. Whether it's rock climbing, yoga, or Pilates, the local sports or leisure centre often offers an array of activities. The beauty of this approach is that you might discover a newfound passion, or at the very least, realize you're ready for a change. The social aspect of pursuing a hobby can also contribute significantly to mental well-being.

Four: The Natural Approach – Go for a Walk

Embrace the natural approach—take a walk. All the benefits of jogging without the sweat and knee strain. Walking offers diverse possibilities: stride to the shops, enjoy nature on a sunny day, or relish an early morning stroll before the day unfolds. Ten minutes of brisk pacing can yield considerable benefits.[47]

Five: The Invisible Approach – Incorporate Exercise into Daily Life

The invisible approach involves incorporating exercise into daily life—gardening, housework, walking or cycling for commuting, opting for stairs over the elevator, and choosing the furthest parking spot. Keeping a record ensures that we meet the weekly exercise quota, and over time, we may find ourselves naturally exceeding it, a truly uplifting realization.

---

[47] 'Mental Health Foundation', How to look after your mental health using exercise (Web Page) < https://www.mentalhealth.org.uk/explore-mental-health/publications/how-look-after-your-mental-health-using-exercise >.

Six: The Competitive Approach – Play Sport

Engage in the competitive approach—play sport. For many, the social benefits of sports become an added bonus. Whether it's the leisurely pace of bowls or the dynamism of tennis, football, netball, or cricket, joining a club offers both physical and social advantages. Playing sports is an excellent way to derive enjoyment from exercise, especially for those with a competitive streak.

Seven: The Companion Approach – Get a Dog

Consider the companion approach—get a dog. Owning a dog necessitates daily walks, providing a triple whammy of exercise, love, and responsibility. If circumstances limit pet ownership, a creative solution like weekend dog walking can turn exercise into a rewarding side hustle.

Finding a Friend or Group – The Social Element of Exercise

Pairing up with a friend or joining a group enhances the social aspect of exercise. Whether it's a walk, a swim, or a sports activity, having a companion makes it more enjoyable and increases the likelihood of sticking to the routine. The social commitment also makes it harder to cancel plans, fostering consistency.

Volunteering – A Holistic Approach to Exercise and Community Support

Volunteering not only provides exercise, but also boosts self-esteem by contributing to the local community. Libraries, doctor's surgeries, and community centres are excellent starting points to identify volunteer opportunities. This dual-purpose activity combines physical exertion with social interaction, fostering a sense of community and creating opportunities for meaningful friendships.

As we immerse ourselves in our newfound exercise routine—those brisk walks, the club memberships, the volunteer work, and the rejuvenation of our gardens—we begin to witness the transformation within ourselves. A couple of walks per week expose us to the benefits of vitamin D,[48] joining clubs or taking up sports introduces us to a network of new friends, and volunteering for the local food bank adds a sense of purpose to our endeavours. The visual and physical improvements in our living spaces contribute to our overall happiness. Our bodies, too, respond positively to this new way of life, and we find ourselves investing three to four hours a week in enjoyable, health-boosting activities.

---

[48]'Medical News Today', Vitamin D: Benefits, deficiency, sources, and dosage (Web Page) <https://www.medicalnewstoday.com/articles/161618>.

However, not everyone in our circles has embraced this journey with the same zeal. There's a lingering 'friend' who consistently finds reasons to opt-out. Too much work, no time, a general lack of enthusiasm—these are the familiar refrains. It's not entirely surprising, we gently suggest to them, as they're missing out on the emotional benefits of exercise.

The promise of doing it later is met with scepticism. In our intimate space—just you, me (apologies, your 'friend'), and this book—honesty prevails. If we can't be forthright here, where can we? Will they truly do it later?

Commencing an exercise regime is admittedly not a walk in the park. If it were, we'd all be seasoned exercisers by now. The reality is, exercise is not the easy option we wish it were. Nonetheless, when it comes to our mental health, the case for exercise is irrefutable. Keeping this unequivocal truth in mind, let's recap the key points we've aimed to convey in this chapter:

1. **Finding Ways to Exercise is Easier Than Perceived** – Contrary to common belief, discovering ways to incorporate exercise into our lives is more feasible than we often admit to ourselves.
2. **A Little Goes a Long Way** – We don't need to undertake Herculean efforts to reap mental and physical benefits from exercise. Even a modest investment yields significant returns.
3. **Social Exercise Enhances Emotional Well-being** – Engaging in exercise as a social activity amplifies its emotional benefits. The camaraderie and shared experiences elevate the overall impact on mental health.
4. **Pleasure Fuels Consistency** – Initiated into the world of exercise, we quickly find pleasure in it. This newfound enjoyment becomes the driving force that sustains our commitment.
5. **Exercise Sparks a Desire for More** – Instead of being a chore, exercise evolves into a desire. The initial steps pave the way for a journey, where the more we exercise, the more we want to exercise.

As emphasized earlier, exercise isn't merely a fleeting benefit; it's the enduring emotional health benefit that keeps on giving. So, let's embrace the joy, the camaraderie, and the countless rewards that accompany our commitment to a healthier, more active lifestyle. The journey is not just about exercise; it's about the profound impact it has on our mental well-being, making each step forward a celebration of our commitment to a happier and healthier self.

Sleep, Brain Work and Art – Balm for the Mind

'Sleep is that golden chain that ties health and our bodies together'
Thomas Dekker[49]

Embarking on the latter half of this concise book, two pivotal insights crystalize. Firstly, there exists a multitude of actions that not only can but should be undertaken to enhance our mental health. Secondly, the benefits derived from these actions are not isolated but intricately intertwined. Whether it's maintaining a healthy diet, engaging in regular exercise, or prioritizing sleep, each element complements and elevates the others, forming a comprehensive strategy for the enhancement and sustenance of mental well-being.

The third indispensable component in our arsenal is sleep. The intricate dance between sleep and mental health unfolds as a dilemma: poor sleep contributes to compromised mental well-being, and in turn, struggling mental health disrupts the ability to achieve restful sleep. This cyclic interplay underscores the complex relationship between the two. Scientific endeavours to unravel the mysteries of the sleeping brain persist, revealing a variety of activities during sleep. Some elevate brain activity, while others reduce it. Crucially, it's during sleep that the brain processes and assimilates positive emotional experiences,[50] playing a pivotal role in our happiness, self-esteem, outlook, and interpersonal connections. Conversely, the deprivation of sleep hampers this process, leading to diminished happiness, lower self-esteem, and an increased susceptibility to mental illness.

The importance of sleep extends beyond its impact on mental well-being. Understanding sleep as a bodily process reveals its various types, including REM (rapid eye movement) sleep,[51] a phase of profound rest.[52] During REM sleep, our brains are most active, processing positive emotional experiences crucial for emotional stability.[53] Failure in this process is believed to heighten susceptibility to suicidal thoughts.[54] While lack of sleep may not be a direct precursor to suicidal tendencies,[55] those grappling with such thoughts often experience sleep disturbances. Hence, sleep emerges not only as a mood enhancer but also as a potential lifesaver.

---

[49]'Thomas Dekker', Thomas Dekker Quotes (Web Page) <https://www.goodreads.com/author/quotes/22587.Thomas_Dekker>
[50]'Eric Suni', Mental Health and Sleep (Web Page) < https://www.sleepfoundation.org/mental-health>.
[51]Ibid.
[52]Ibid.
[53]Ibid.
[54]Ibid.
[55]Ibid.

The pervasive influence of our modern, gadget-laden lives on sleep cannot be overstated. The impact of electronic devices on our sleep is intricately tied to, our circadian rhythms,[56] the natural cycles dictated by our biological clocks.[57] These clocks, composed of proteins,[58] orchestrate our circadian rhythms,[59] regulating functions such as the release of melatonin,[60] our 'drowsy' hormone,[61] ensuring we sleep at night and stay awake during the day.[62]

The prevalent use of electronic devices, emitting blue light, disrupts this delicate balance. Blue light stimulates the brain, contradicting the circadian rhythm's signal to sleep. Consequently, sleep patterns are compromised. However, the narrative extends beyond the negative impact. Strategic exposure to blue light during the day can realign circadian rhythms, enhancing alertness during waking hours and promoting relaxation at night, facilitating better sleep. Although caution is advised about electronic use close to bedtime, daytime utilization might even yield benefits for sleep patterns.

Electronic devices, particularly laptops, phones, and TVs, often expose us to blue light. This light acts as a stimulant, conflicting with our circadian rhythm's sleep signals. Yet, this is only part of the story, as blue light can also assist in resetting circadian rhythms,[63] optimizing alertness during the day and relaxation at night,[64] thus facilitating better sleep.[65] While excessive use of electronic devices may trigger headaches, or contribute to feelings of isolation, these effects vary individually. Reports on the negative mental health impacts of electronic use should be scrutinised for evidence and reliability, rather than succumbing to sensationalism.

Despite the complexities surrounding electronic device use, the paramount importance of sleep remains unaltered. Optimal sleep is more likely when coupled with physical fitness and a well-balanced diet, steering clear of heavy or late-night meals. Caffeine and alcohol, recognized impediments to sleep, should be consumed judiciously.

Once again, the intricate web linking mental well-being, diet, exercise, and sleep is unmistakable. These elements synergize, creating a holistic approach to mental health. As we navigate

---

[56]'National Institute of General Medical Sciences', Circadian Rhythms (Web Page) <https://bilimblogum.wordpress.com/wp-content/uploads/2022/11/fact-sheet-circadian-rhythms.pdf>.
[57]Ibid.
[58]Ibid.
[59]'National Institute of General Medical Sciences', Circadian Rhythms (Web Page) <https://bilimblogum.wordpress.com/wp-content/uploads/2022/11/fact-sheet-circadian-rhythms.pdf>.
[60]Ibid.
[61]Ibid.
[62]Ibid.
[63]'Rob Newsom', Blue Light: what it is and how it affects sleep (Web Page) <https://www.sleepfoundation.org/bedroom-environment/blue-light>.
[64]Ibid.
[65]Ibid.

the intricacy of factors influencing our well-being, it becomes evident that addressing each facet—diet, exercise, and sleep—in harmony is the key to unlocking a healthier, more resilient mind.

The societal landscape, dominated by electronic devices, has irrevocably altered our relationship with sleep. The digital age, marked by the constant hum of notifications, the glow of screens, and the accessibility of information, has introduced new challenges to achieving restful sleep. Yet, the narrative around the impact of electronic devices on our mental well-being often lacks subtlety.

The circadian rhythms that govern our sleep-wake cycle are deeply ingrained in our biological makeup. These rhythms dictate our natural physical, behavioural, and mental cycles, ensuring our bodies respond to light, guiding us to sleep at night and remain awake during the day. At the core of this regulation lies melatonin, the hormone responsible for inducing drowsiness and preparing the body for sleep.

However, the prevalence of electronic devices, such as laptops, phones, and TVs, introduces a complicating factor—blue light. Emitting a stimulating form of light, blue light acts as a wakefulness promoter, contradicting the circadian rhythm's cues for bedtime. This disruption in the delicate balance of our internal clocks leads to compromised sleep patterns.

Nevertheless, the story of electronic devices and sleep is not one-dimensional. Blue light exposure can be strategic; its impact varies depending on the timing of exposure. While nighttime use may hinder sleep, daytime exposure can assist in resetting circadian rhythms, enhancing alertness during waking hours, and contributing to better sleep quality at night.

Acknowledging the negative impact of excessive electronic device use on sleep is imperative. Headaches triggered by prolonged screen time and the potential for social isolation due to excessive smartphone use are valid concerns. However, these effects are nuanced and individualized, often stemming from misuse rather than inherent characteristics of electronic devices.

The narrative surrounding electronic devices and mental health often carries a sensationalized tone. Reports of detrimental impacts on mental well-being should be critically examined, separating evidence-based claims from sensationalism. While acknowledging potential negative outcomes, it's essential to recognize that responsible use of electronic devices, coupled with awareness and moderation, can mitigate these risks.

The intricate interplay between mental well-being, diet, exercise, and sleep persists as a recurrent theme. Each element of this quartet contributes to the overall fabric of our mental health.

Just as a symphony requires harmony among its instruments, our mental well-being thrives when these components are in sync.

Returning to the fundamental importance of sleep, it's evident that achieving optimal rest is intricately linked to physical fitness and dietary habits. A well-rested body, devoid of aches and pains, coupled with efficient respiratory function, is more conducive to quality sleep. Moreover, mindful consumption—avoiding heavy or late-night meals, moderating caffeine intake, and being cautious with alcohol—further supports the quest for restful sleep.

In the intricate dance of mental well-being, where diet, exercise, and sleep are partners, the subtleties of electronic device use come into focus. While acknowledging the challenges posed by the digital age, it's crucial to distinguish between the potential benefits and drawbacks of electronic devices. Responsible usage, informed by an understanding of circadian rhythms, can transform these devices from adversaries into allies in the pursuit of a well-balanced, resilient mind.

In conclusion, the symbiotic relationship between mental well-being, diet, exercise, and sleep remains an undeniable truth. As we navigate the riddle of factors influencing our mental health, it becomes clear that a holistic approach, addressing each facet with intention and balance, is the key to fostering a resilient and flourishing mind. Just as knitting mends the 'ravelled sleeve of care,' tending to the interconnected elements of our well-being can weave a fabric of strength and vitality for the mind.

Nurturing Mental Well-being: The Cognitive Symphony of Brain Exercise and Literary Escape

The question lingers: can a workout for the brain truly contribute to our mental health? Anecdotal evidence seems to support the idea, but the scientific community remains divided on this matter. Extensive research investigates into the benefits of brain gym activities, yielding mixed conclusions.[66] On one side are sceptics who dismiss brain exercises as mere commercial ploys, aimed at parting us from our hard-earned money or subjecting us to online advertising. On the other side are those who acknowledge some benefits but question whether these outweigh the potential downsides, such as tiredness, stress, or frustration. Despite the debate, the primary advantage of brain exercises often revolve around cognitive function improvement and enhanced memory. These, in turn, indirectly elevate mental health by boosting self-esteem, sharpening thought processes, and enhancing concentration.

---

[66]'Kendra Cherry', How you can strengthen your brain with exercises (Web Page) <https://www.verywellmind.com/brain-exercises-to-strengthen-your-mind-2795039>.

Yet, there is another facet to these activities—they are enjoyable. Brain exercises need not be expensive; newspapers frequently feature crosswords and puzzle pages. Engaging in games like chess or bridge, or even playing board games, can be both mentally stimulating and socially enriching. The joy derived from these activities contributes to mental well-being.

For those seeking a solo mental health boost, reading stands out as a powerful ally. The genre matters less than the act itself, as the primary goal is relaxation and enjoyment. Whether diving into the latest John Grisham novel, immersing oneself in Jane Austen's world, exploring the history of big trucks, or digging into the Sunday Magazine, the act of reading significantly benefits mental health. Reading serves as an escape, allowing individuals to immerse themselves in alternative worlds, temporarily freeing them from the stresses of daily life. While all forms of reading offer cognitive benefits, fiction emerges as a potent genre. Research suggests that the mental health advantages of reading are extensive, leading to the emergence of bibliotherapy as a treatment for depression, involving copious amounts of reading and discussion.[67]

The benefits of reading extend beyond cognitive enhancements; fiction reading, in particular, nurtures empathy. Strengthening empathy fosters healthier relationships, filled with associated mental health advantages. The term 'narrative absorption' describes the deep immersion into a story,[68] believed to induce higher levels of meaningful contemplation.[69] Some studies even propose that reading fiction activates the prefrontal cortex,[70] enhancing our ability to perceive actions in perspective.[71] This is particularly pertinent for young individuals, such as teens and young adults, as the prefrontal cortex develops more slowly than the rest of the brain. Maintaining perspective is crucial for mental well-being, as a loss of it can magnify everyday problems to seemingly insurmountable levels. A well-crafted fiction story can even stave off depression for months, lingering in its positive effects long after the final chapter concludes.[72]

In navigating the realm of brain exercises and literary escapades, the overarching theme remains clear: the pursuit of mental well-being is a multifaceted journey. The symphony of brain exercises and reading, when harmonized, contributes to a holistic approach to mental health. Just as a well-coordinated orchestra produces a melodious composition, engaging in brain exercises and indulging in the immersive world of literature weaves a masterpiece of cognitive resilience and emotional vitality.

---

[67]'Richard Sima', *The mental health benefits of reading* (Web Page) <https://www.psychologytoday.com/us/blog/the-art-effect/202203/the-mental-health-benefits-reading>.
[68]Ibid.
[69]Ibid.
[70]Ibid.
[71]Ibid.
[72]Ibid.

As we explore the realms of brain gym activities and literary retreats, it becomes evident that the integration of these elements into our lives can yield profound benefits for mental health. The complexities and distinctions of these practices provide a rich landscape for individual exploration and personal growth. Just as the 'ravelled sleeve of care' is knitted up through the interplay of various threads, so too is mental well-being nurtured through the interconnected dance of brain exercise and literary engagement.

Broaden Your Horizons: The Mental Health Benefits of Skill Acquisition

Seeking a new qualification, whether academic or practical, opens avenues for personal and mental growth. While the prospect of further study may not initially create images of literary indulgence, the benefits extend far beyond the confines of books. Engaging in such self-advancement not only offers a mental challenge but also fosters self-esteem through academic achievements. Additionally, the social benefits of interacting with new people can be significant, if there is a safe environment.

Embarking on a journey of acquiring a new qualification provides a unique mental challenge, stimulating the brain in novel ways. This mental exercise contributes to cognitive well-being, enhancing our ability to navigate complexities and think critically. The process of learning, irrespective of the subject matter, cultivates mental resilience, preparing us to face challenges with a more adaptable mindset.

The boost to self-esteem accompanying academic success is a noteworthy mental health benefit. Achieving milestones in the pursuit of a qualification reinforces our sense of capability and accomplishment. This newfound confidence goes beyond the academic realm, permeating other aspects of life and providing a buffer against stress and uncertainty.

Furthermore, the social dimension of further study plays a pivotal role in enhancing mental well-being. Engaging with fellow learners, whether in person or through online platforms, provides opportunities for meaningful connections. Even virtual courses facilitate idea-sharing and often include face-to-face gatherings, fostering a sense of community. These interactions not only broaden our social circles but also introduce shared experiences, creating a common ground for conversation. Awkward moments of establishing connections are mitigated as conversations naturally revolve around the shared pursuit of knowledge.

Online courses, in particular, offer a wealth of opportunities for social stimulation. Collaborative discussions, group projects, and forums create a vibrant learning environment where individuals can exchange ideas and perspectives. The shared commitment to educational advancement serves as a powerful catalyst for building friendships and networks.

The potential career opportunities arising from acquiring a new qualification contribute to emotional balance, especially in times of pressure or change. A qualification may open doors to different career paths or provide a fresh perspective, offering a sense of purpose and direction. The mental well-being associated with career satisfaction and growth is invaluable, impacting overall life satisfaction.

However, self-advancement need not be confined to academic pursuits. Acquiring practical skills, such as decorating or plumbing, can yield a sense of self-confidence and accomplishment. The ability to apply newly acquired DIY (do it yourself) skills not only saves money but also instils a sense of empowerment. Engaging in hands-on activities fosters a connection between the mind and the physical world, promoting a holistic approach to mental well-being.

Moreover, pursuing a hobby is another avenue for mental nourishment. Whether it's cultivating a garden, learning a musical instrument, or exploring artistic endeavours, hobbies provide a satisfying outlet for creativity and personal expression. The sense of achievement derived from honing a skill or completing a project contributes positively to mental health.

In conclusion, the decision to pursue a new qualification, whether academic or practical, is a transformative journey with multifaceted benefits for mental well-being. The mental challenge, enhanced self-esteem, and social interactions inherent in such pursuits create a holistic approach to personal and cognitive growth. Whether through academic endeavours, practical skills acquisition, or engaging in hobbies, the path to self-advancement opens doors to a more enriched and resilient mental state.

Mandala Therapy: Colouring Your Way to Serenity

Amidst emerging trends, a profoundly beneficial hobby entices—adult colouring books featuring intricate mandala designs. Mandala art involves intricate patterns waiting to be infused with colour, offering a unique avenue for focusing on mental health and well-being. Science emphasizes the therapeutic impact of creative acts, particularly in stimulating the right side of the brain, responsible for problem-solving and thinking outside the box—essential tools for navigating the stresses of daily life. The repetitive nature of colouring itself contributes to a sense of calmness, even reducing heart rate and allowing the tensions of the day to dissipate, fostering good mental health.

Engaging in adult colouring books, however, may pose a hurdle as it's often perceived as a childish activity. Contrary to this misconception, adult colouring books bear little resemblance to their child-oriented counterparts. While both children and adults benefit from the calming effects of repetitive and creative colouring, the objectives and designs differ significantly. A child's colouring book aims to teach about colours and develop dexterity, while an adult colouring book is meticulously crafted to stimulate creativity and provide a source of calm and relaxation.

Drawing a parallel, one might consider a child riding a toy car versus an adult driving a real one—both involve a 'car,' but the purposes and experiences vastly differ. Similarly, the act of colouring, especially intricate mandalas, transforms into a meditative and soothing practice for adults. For those grappling with stress, unable to escape the pressures of work, relationships, or the daily commute, adult colouring proves to be a worthwhile endeavour. With the minimal investment of a colouring book and a set of pencils, this activity presents an experiment with little downside and potentially profound benefits.

The intricate designs of mandalas provide a canvas for creative expression and exploration. The act of colouring within these complex patterns becomes a therapeutic journey, allowing the mind to focus, unwind, and escape the demands of the external world. The colours chosen, the strokes applied, and the rhythmic repetition all contribute to a mindful and immersive experience. As the hues fill the intricate spaces, a sense of accomplishment and tranquillity unfolds.

Scientifically, the impact of such creative pursuits extends beyond the immediate meditative benefits. The stimulation of the right side of the brain during colouring enhances problem-solving skills and encourages innovative thinking. This mental exercise becomes a powerful tool in combating the cognitive challenges posed by modern life.

In essence, adult colouring books, particularly those featuring mandalas, offer a gateway to a serene and creative realm. Shedding preconceived notions of childhood associations, adults can embrace this activity as a mindful practice, a form of art therapy that transcends the ordinary and nurtures mental well-being. So, for those seeking an affordable and accessible experiment in self-care, the world of adult colouring books stands ready to unfold, inviting individuals to embark on a journey of creativity, tranquillity, and holistic mental rejuvenation.

Unleashing Creativity for Mental Wellness

Beyond the routine of daily life lies a realm of creative outlets that can significantly contribute to our mental health. Engaging with music, theatre, films, or TV series not only stimulates our brains but also presents opportunities for social interaction. Sharing thoughts on the latest cliff-hanger with friends or colleagues fosters a sense of community and connection. Music, in particular, emerges as a powerful tool in reducing stress and promoting relaxation.

Music, with its diverse genres and melodies, is thought to have a profound impact on our well-being. It regulates the release of cortisol, the 'fight or flight' hormone, lowers heart rate, and triggers the release of endorphins, the feel-good neurotransmitters. Music serves as a distraction that allows our minds to process emotions, leading to an improved sense of perspective. The type of music that brings relaxation is subjective; what matters is finding the tunes that resonate with individual preferences. Whether it's calming sounds for sleep or the energizing beats of heavy metal, the key is to embrace what works uniquely for each person.

White noise, a form of repetitive and relaxing sounds, offers another auditory avenue to calmness, especially when seeking better sleep. Various apps on our phones provide a range of white noise options, from the hum of an aircraft to the soothing rhythm of a washing machine, catering to diverse preferences and aiding many in achieving a tranquil state.

For those seeking a more active form of participation, venturing into the world of visual arts can be immensely rewarding. Adult colouring books, as discussed earlier, offer a taste of the creative process, but why not explore full-scale art? Painting, drawing, sketching, pottery, or sculpture—each form provides a unique channel for self-expression. The undeniable benefits of these activities stem from the relaxation they offer to the brain.

Much like the meditative practice of colouring mandalas, engaging in art stimulates the right side of the brain, contributing to enhanced perspective and problem-solving abilities. The act of creating art becomes a therapeutic journey, allowing individuals to explore their thoughts, emotions, and creativity. Whether it's through the strokes of a paintbrush or the moulding of clay, the process itself becomes a form of mindfulness, grounding individuals in the present moment.

The beauty of these creative pursuits lies in their adaptability to individual preferences and needs. Each person can carve their path to mental wellness through the artistic expressions that resonate with them. The key is to embrace the creative process as a means of self-discovery and a tool for nurturing mental health.

In conclusion, the avenues to stimulate the creative side of our brains are vast and diverse. Whether through the auditory enchantment of music, the communal experience of theatre or film, or the hands-on exploration of visual arts, each creative outlet contributes to mental well-being in its unique way. The pursuit of creativity becomes a personal journey, a canvas painted with the threads of self-expression, relaxation, and enhanced cognitive function.

Physical Bliss: The Power of Massage

Unlocking the potential of our physical bodies can trigger the release of endorphins, providing a natural high and promoting mental well-being. A massage, beyond its muscle-soothing benefits, proves to be a holistic method for calming and relaxation. While not suitable for everyone, as some may not be comfortable with touch, for those who relish the sensation, there is a diverse range of massages available.

From deeply invigorating sessions to gentle and soothing experiences, massages cater to various preferences. For those not keen on intense muscle manipulation, a tranquil head massage offers a pleasing alternative. On the flip side, indulging in a foot massage provides a rejuvenating experience at the other end of the spectrum. The key lies in finding the right type of massage that aligns with personal comfort and preferences, unlocking the physical pathway to mental rejuvenation.

Embracing Nature's Tranquillity

Integrating nature into our daily lives can be a simple yet powerful way to enhance mental well-being. Placing a bird feeder in the backyard or on the terrace invites moments of relaxation as we observe the rhythmic dance of birds feeding, fluttering to and from the food source, and indulging in the seeds and nuts provided.

This chapter emphasizes that various avenues exist for nurturing mental health, combining cognitive stimulation and relaxation. The key lies in discovering what resonates with each individual. Whether it's the serene act of lounging on the sofa, immersing oneself in a captivating book with a glass of red wine in hand, or engaging in a hobby like woodwork, stargazing, or writing – each is a cause for celebration. For those inclined towards communal experiences, group activities such as night school or online qualifications can invigorate the mind.

There is no one-size-fits-all solution; the multitude of options available allows individuals to preserve and improve their mental well-being in ways that align with their unique preferences. The essence is to find that perfect harmony between cognitive stimulation and relaxation, embracing the diverse opportunities that nature and personal interests offer for a holistic approach to mental wellness.

Mates, Mindfulness and Maintaining Balance

'Friends are the family you choose'
Jess C. Scott[73]

In this concluding chapter, our focus widens to encompass a more comprehensive exploration of actions that contribute to our overall well-being. We explore into the realms of friendships, attitudes, and the invaluable practice of mindfulness. By now, it should be apparent that the symbiotic relationship between physical and mental health is a recurring theme throughout our journey. The narrative consistently highlights the significance of social interaction, making it a convenient point to initiate our discussion.

Cultivating Meaningful Connections – Unveiling the Dynamics of the Law of Attraction

The concept of the law of attraction, often propelled by the currents of social media, emerges as a compelling force in our lives. While scrutinizing it reveals refined complexities, adopting a broad perspective acknowledges its merits. Viewing it as a theoretical framework from which valuable lessons can be extracted, we discover that living by its message isn't obligatory, but rather an option.

At its core, the law of attraction posits that we gravitate towards individuals who mirror aspects of our own nature. As we spend more time in their company, a reciprocal interaction takes root, shaping both parties involved. The traits initially drawing us together gain prominence, leading to either the vortex of a detrimental cycle or the virtues of a beneficial one. If the initial connection is rooted in negativity, our propensity for negative thinking solidifies, fostering a relationship that thrives on criticism. Conversely, if shared joy forms the foundation, our collective outlook on life is enriched by the positivity we collectively embrace.

Consider a scenario: a bustling coffee shop during our lunch break, a spare seat at a colleague's table, and a nod of invitation. A new friendship begins, triggered by a mention of a positive event—a new, flexible, and friendly boss. This sparks a conversation that extends to shared interests in sports, art, or other pursuits. The camaraderie grows, leading to invitations to events and the formation of a circle of friends who share a positive outlook on life. The men-

---

[73]'Jess C Scott', Jess C Scott Quotes (Web Page) <https://www.wisdomtimes.com/quotes/author/jess-c-scott/>.

tal well-being benefits become apparent as optimism becomes a driving force, influencing not only our thoughts but also our physical well-being through healthier habits.

On the contrary, envision a different narrative: the same coffee shop, the same colleague, a gloomy conversation about unfavourable weather and a critical perspective on the new boss. The negativity perpetuates, influencing subsequent encounters and shaping a social circle centred around pessimism and discontent. This contrast underscores the profound impact of our connections on our well-being.

The Power of Social Bonds and the Complexities of the Law of Attraction

Building social connections emerges as a cornerstone in enhancing our mental health, with the law of attraction serving as a guiding principle to navigate this terrain positively. While the concept may seem simplistic, it holds merit in our tendency to be drawn to like-minded individuals and, in doing so, reinforcing shared traits. The key takeaway lies in our ability to catalyse positive change in those with negative outlooks by embodying positivity ourselves. Whether they absorb the message or not, our path may diverge, but the effort remains worthwhile. Smiling, minimizing complaints (though occasional grumbling is a universal indulgence), and focusing on the positives attract friendships with other optimistic individuals, creating a cycle of upbeat discussions and activities that elevate our mental well-being.

Cultivating Gratitude – A Radiant Beacon in Life's Journey

Consider the podcast 'You, Me and the Big C', a poignant exploration of living with terminal cancer by three resilient women—Deborah James, Lauren Mahon, and Rachel Bland. Despite facing an unimaginably desperate situation, their approach is remarkably upbeat, emphasizing the importance of living fully with the time they have. While not every moment is optimistic, the podcast serves as a testament to finding gratitude amidst adversity.

Reflecting on this, we realize that even in our own lives, there are numerous things for which we can be grateful. Shifting our outlook involves consciously concentrating on these positives and leaving behind the negatives. For those who find this challenging, maintaining a gratitude journal can be transformative. Record five events each day that bring gratitude or happiness—an encounter with waddling geese, a considerate driver, an unexpected cup of coffee from a colleague, a favourite snack, a call to a loved one, or the comforting presence of a purring cat. These seemingly trivial occurrences, when acknowledged and documented, accumulate to create a record of goodness in our lives, fostering an enduring sense of well-being. Life, upon closer inspection, is a collection of such moments—easy to overlook but collectively shaping a narrative that is undeniably positive. Let's not only think about it but also jot it down, ensuring we remember and cherish the beauty in the everyday.

Mastering the Art of Mindfulness for Well-Being

The term 'mindfulness' permeates contemporary discourse, although its origins trace back to Buddhism,[74] encapsulating the ability to dwell in the present moment.[75] This practice aspires to heighten awareness,[76] instil calmness,[77] and maintain perspective,[78] urging us to extend kindness to ourselves—an aspect often overlooked in our daily lives.[79] The chapter revisits this crucial characteristic later, underscoring mindfulness as a tool to confront challenging thoughts and, notably, alleviate stress. While not universally effective, it stands as a technique worthy of exploration for navigating the strains of daily existence. As with any skill, mindfulness demands effort and practice to master.

By immersing ourselves in the present, we gradually unravel the intricacies of how thoughts permeate our minds, paving the way for better control over their entry. However, the challenge lies in the baggage many carry—past traumas, experiences of abuse, or the lingering effects of bereavement. The impact of such crisis points, termed 'psychological trauma' by Janet's French psychodynamic school,[80] can fracture our mental cohesiveness,[81] leaving enduring scars. It's important to acknowledge that a brief exploration of mindfulness cannot offer comprehensive solutions for these profound challenges. Serious situations may necessitate medical or psychological intervention, with counselling emerging as a valuable tool, provided full commitment is given to the process. Medication, under the guidance of qualified practitioners, is also a potential avenue.

The complexity of mental health, as highlighted by Engel's model from 1981,[82] and more recent studies like Ruini and Cesetti's in 2020, highlights the evolving understanding of the field. While acknowledging the absence of definitive answers, mindfulness emerges as a potential

---

[74]'Sonya Matejko', What's the background of mindfulness? (Web Page) <https://psychcentral.com/lib/a-brief-history-of-mindfulness-in-the-usa-and-its-impact-on-our-lives>.
[75]Ibid.
[76]Ibid.
[77]Ibid.
[78]Ibid.
[79]'Mind', Mindfulness (Web Page) <https://www.mind.org.uk/information-support/drugs-and-treatments/mindfulness/about-mindfulness/>.
[80]Giulio Perrotta, 'Psychological Trauma: Definition, Clinical Contexts, Neural Correlations and Therapeutic Approaches Recent Discoveries' [2019] (1) Current Research in Psychiatry and Brain Disorders 1.
[81]Ibid.
[82]George L. Engel, 'The Clinical Application of the Biopsychosocial Model' (1981) 6(2) The Journal of Medicine and Philosophy: A Forum for Bioethics and Philosophy of Medicine 101.

aid, if not a panacea, for mental stress. It equips us to intercept negative thoughts about the past or future, enabling us to control, if not eradicate, their influence on our identity. The second facet of mindfulness involves decoding the language of our bodies—a physical dimension where stress, mood swings, and anxiety manifest. Early recognition empowers us to address these issues before they dig in themselves.

Crucially, mindfulness encourages creating a space between negative thoughts and our current existence. This distance fosters the ability to rationalize intruding thoughts, contextualize them, and mount a counteraction. While mindfulness is promoted for its day-to-day benefits, evidence suggests its potential efficacy in managing depression, anxiety, and stress. It may even extend its benefits to deeper-seated mental illnesses. However, attempting to teach mindfulness within the confines of this book would do it an injustice, for it's a profound technique that demands time, patience, and dedicated practice.

Numerous resources, including books, websites, and courses, are readily available to those willing to explore mindfulness. Yet, the true challenge lies in committing to the process, trusting in its transformative power, and understanding that becoming a more mindful person is a journey requiring commitment. It may not happen overnight, but the rewards—both enjoyable and profoundly beneficial for our well-being—are well worth the effort.

Cultivating Self-Awareness for Personal Empowerment

An invaluable outcome of mindfulness is the heightened self-awareness it bestows. This concept encompasses two key dimensions.[83] Firstly, it involves the ability to objectively observe our actions and thoughts,[84] fostering a near-dispassionate analysis of our behaviours.[85] Importantly, this doesn't advocate for every action to be coldly calculated;[86] rather, it encourages an understanding of the motivations behind our actions and thoughts.[87] The second facet of self-awareness involves recognizing the impact of our actions, feelings, and thoughts on those in our immediate surroundings us.[88]

Identifying a lack of self-awareness is often easier than defining the concept itself. Signs of a deficiency include emotions spiralling out of control, difficulty being accountable for one's ac-

---

[83] Erin Heger and John Mutziger, '4 reasons why self-awareness matters and 3 ways to develop it' (Media Release, 20 January 2022) <https://www.businessinsider.nl/4-reasons-why-self-awareness-matters-and-3-ways-to-develop-it/>.
[84] Erin Heger and John Mutziger, '4 reasons why self-awareness matters and 3 ways to develop it' (Media Release, 20 January 2022) <https://www.businessinsider.nl/4-reasons-why-self-awareness-matters-and-3-ways-to-develop-it/>.
[85] Ibid.
[86] Ibid.
[87] Ibid.
[88] Ibid.

tions, acting without consideration for others, and a sense of automatism in navigating life. The journey toward self-awareness isn't facile; it necessitates training and a willingness to invest time in honing this skill. Mindfulness serves as an initial step, facilitating the development of the ability to introspect and fostering the empathy essential for understanding how others perceive us.

In a society where human interactions are fundamental to emotional well-being, dismissing concern about others' perceptions may be misguided. Even those who profess indifference to others' opinions might benefit from introspection. Micro-reflection,[89] a daily practice of spending a few minutes journaling about successes,[90] areas for improvement,[91] and strategies for the future,[92] serves as a practical tool to enhance self-awareness.

Another avenue for development lies in seeking external perspectives. Candid conversations with family, friends, and colleagues, especially those not considered close friends, can offer valuable insights. Feedback, even when delivered with the intention of constructive criticism, contributes to self-awareness. Therapy, such as counselling or participation in group activities, presents an expedited route for those deeply committed to cultivating self-awareness. Emotional awareness workshops, in particular, can yield substantial rewards.

While embracing the path to self-awareness, one must acknowledge that change is a constant, rendering self-awareness an ongoing skill that requires continual reinforcement. Recognition of daily actions guided by personal values, awareness of strengths and weaknesses in various situations, and understanding the impact on those around us signify attainment of self-awareness.

The rewards of self-awareness are infinite. Foremost, it fosters flourishing self-esteem and pride in one's authentic actions and thoughts. Self-acceptance becomes the bedrock, alleviating social stresses, enhancing relationships, and even benefiting professional endeavours through increased confidence and a heightened understanding of how others perceive us. Social anxiety diminishes as self-awareness empowers individuals to navigate potential misinterpretations of their actions. For instance, in the workplace, a self-aware person can modify behaviour based on an understanding of how their actions may be perceived by colleagues.

As self-awareness grows, confidence flourishes, anxiety recedes, and self-growth becomes inevitable. Confidence is bolstered through proactive decision-making, creating a virtuous circle where increased self-esteem perpetuates ongoing personal development. Ultimately,

---

[89]Tasha Eichenseher, 'How to develop self-awareness and why it's important' (Media Release, 21 April 2022) < https://psychcentral.com/health/self-awareness >.
[90]Ibid.
[91]Ibid.
[92]Ibid.

self-awareness stands as a virtuous circle, continuously nurturing personal empowerment and well-being.

Navigating Decision-Making: Embracing Deliberation Over Overthinking

The ability to make decisions swiftly and stick to them might seem enviable, alleviating the agony of pondering whether to attend a party or stay home. Yet is the process of overthinking, plagued by considerations and weighing pros and cons, truly a curse? Complex decisions, such as changing jobs or moving homes, demand thorough contemplation. The production of lists detailing advantages and disadvantages may not offer immediate clarity, but does that render overthinking inherently detrimental?

In reality, very few decisions in life benefit from impulsivity. The issue with overthinking doesn't lie in the act itself but in society's peculiar disposition toward those who take their time to arrive at a decision. There exists a romanticized notion that impulsiveness, living or dying by instinctive reactions, holds greater value than measured, reasoned conclusions. This perspective, epitomized in Rudyard Kipling's poem 'If', suggests admiration for those who can whimsically toss away their fortune and then recover. However, this idealized view is outdated and rooted in social engineering—a tool used by the ruling classes to maintain control.

The hero in 'If' possesses the backing and security to casually squander a fortune on a whim—an extravagance most individuals lack. Rational decision-making is not a weakness but a strength, and it challenges the antiquated notion that impulsive actions define courage. Some may feel frustrated when grappling with indecision, leading to mental health concerns like anger, diminished self-esteem, and a sense of letting others down. In such instances, a helpful strategy is to brainstorm, jotting down every aspect of the problem and transforming the list into a mind-map—a powerful tool for managing anxiety. The mind-map visually organizes various dilemmas and counterarguments, freeing the mind to concentrate on processing information and determining optimal outcomes.

Society's perception of overthinking as a problem should be reconsidered. Instead, let's reframe it as rational thinking, considered thinking, or balanced thinking. This semantic shift transforms overthinking from a perceived weakness into a recognized strength[93]—one that embraces thoughtful deliberation and rejects impulsive decision-making.[94]

---

[93] Stevan Nikolin et al, 'An investigation of working memory deficits in depression using the n-back task: A systematic review and meta-analysis' (2021) 284 (April) Journal of Affective Disorders 1.
[94] 'Mindmaps.com', What is mind mapping? What are its uses? (Web Page) <https://www.mindmaps.com/what-is-mind-mapping/>.

Understanding PTSD: A Deeper Look at Post-Traumatic Stress Disorder

Anxiety, a pervasive and debilitating mental health condition, is often encapsulated by the term PTSD, or post-traumatic stress disorder. However, in the contemporary discourse, the overuse of this term threatens to dilute the gravity of its implications. Taking a moment to clarify PTSD is essential, as its severity demands recognition.

PTSD emerges from profoundly traumatic experiences,[95] such as war or sexual assault,[96] leaving indelible imprints on the mental well-being of both adults,[97] and, more prevalently, children.[98] This condition induces severe distress and significantly disrupts even routine daily activities.[99] Mundane occurrences can serve as triggers for anxiety, exemplified by war veterans experiencing heightened anxiety upon hearing the backfire of a car exhaust—an often-cited classic example.[100] The consequence is a tendency for individuals with PTSD to withdraw from life, seeking to avoid exposure to anything that might act as a trigger for the disorder. In the scenario mentioned earlier,[101] a military veteran may avoid venturing outside,[102] where the likelihood of encountering a backfiring car is higher.[103]

PTSD is a complex and profound condition that necessitates professional intervention. Its impact extends beyond the immediate aftermath of the traumatic event, permeating daily life and challenging the individual's ability to navigate routine activities without heightened anxiety. The triggers for PTSD can be seemingly innocuous, making it imperative for those affected to seek support and assistance from mental health professionals. Recognizing the gravity of PTSD and acknowledging the need for professional intervention are crucial steps toward supporting individuals grappling with the aftermath of traumatic experiences.

Embracing Balance: A Harmony of Life's Counterweights

In the intricate dance of life, we are continually challenged to find balance—be it in work-life dynamics, emotional stability, or the delicate dance of weighing risks against benefits. This constant balancing act is a fundamental aspect of the human experience, and embracing it as such, transforms the pursuit of balance, from a problem into a natural endeavour.

---

[95]'Jessica Hamblen', What is PTSD? A handout from the National Center for PTSD (Web Page) <http://www.ncptsd.va.gov/ncmain/ncdocs/handouts/handout_What%20is%20PTSD.pdf>.
[96]Ibid.
[97]Ibid.
[98]Ibid.
[99]Ibid.
[100]Ibid.
[101]Ibid.
[102]Ibid.
[103]Ibid.

Extremes, even in seemingly positive attributes like unyielding positivity, can be counterproductive. A perpetual optimist might inadvertently become somewhat irksome; therefore, a more balanced approach, blending enthusiasm with occasional pragmatism, is often more appealing. Similarly, a life dominated solely by work or relentless pleasure-seeking can both have negative repercussions. The key lies in recognising that we require a blend of both—some work and some play, some commitment and some autonomy—to foster a well-rounded existence.

In relationships, an exclusive dedication to a person, while rooted in intense love, can verge on suffocating. Conversely, complete isolation leaves us feeling desolate and alone. The lesson here is that balance is crucial in all facets of life, each person defining it uniquely based on their values and priorities. Striving for balance becomes a tool for promoting physical and mental well-being when we recognize that sweet spot—when we are predominantly happy, settled, and content.

As you conclude this exploration, it's our hope that the insights shared in this book will pave the way for a more achievable sense of balance in the lives, of those who have engaged with its pages. May your journey towards balance, be fulfilling, bringing you moments of happiness, tranquillity, and contentment.

Summing it All Up

*'There is a crack in everything.
That's how the light gets in'*
Leonard Cohen[104]

In our exploration of maintaining optimal mental health, addressing mental health concerns, and understanding the intricate dance between our physical and mental well-being, we have embarked on a journey through the scientific intricacies of mental wellness. Our investigation has probed the profound impact our lifestyle choices wield on the intricate mechanisms of our brains, underscoring the paramount importance of self-awareness in fostering and preserving our mental health.

The overarching narrative is one that radiates positivity and empowerment. By orchestrating incremental adjustments to our lives and reshaping our perspectives on life's challenges, we wield the power to elevate not only our physical but also our mental well-being. While the necessity for professional interventions may arise in certain circumstances, the transformative potential of the changes we can personally instigate often unfolds as a beacon of hope, yielding remarkable improvements in our emotional landscape.

This book encapsulates several key insights, forming the bedrock of a holistic approach to mental and emotional well-being:

The Essential Role of Mental Well-being: Our mental well-being is not merely a peripheral aspect of our existence; it's the linchpin that determines our happiness and our capacity to extract the utmost fulfilment from our lives.

Interconnectedness of Physical and Mental Well-being: The symbiotic relationship between mental and physical well-being is a recurring theme, with positive developments in one realm invariably casting a positive shadow over the other.

Factors Contributing to Emotional Well-being:

a) **Nutrition as Nourishment:** The sustenance we derive from a diverse and healthy diet emerges as a cornerstone. It's not just about meeting dietary requirements, but

---

[104] 'Good Housekeeping', 45 inspirational mental health quotes (Web Page) <https://www.goodhousekeeping.com/life/a39739060/mental-health-quotes/>.

about curating a vibrant palette of fruits, vegetables, nuts, seeds, and the inclusion of omega-3-rich fish, olive oil, and judicious amounts of red meats, dairy, and carbohydrates. Hydration, primarily through water, stands as a non-negotiable component.

b) **Exercise as an Elixir:** The alchemy of at least 150 minutes per week of heart-rate-elevating exercise reveals its transformative potential. Whether through structured gym workouts, the therapeutic embrace of gardening, the rhythmic cadence of housework, or the simple act of walking, exercise becomes a conduit for improved mental health. The communal or partnered aspect of exercise garners special mention, not just for its facilitation of physical activity but for the mental health benefits woven into the fabric of social interaction.

c) **The Pillars of Restful Sleep:** The cornerstone of emotional well-being is anchored in the realm of sleep—regular and sufficient, it provides the much-needed restoration and rejuvenation for our mental faculties.

d) **Brain-stimulating Pursuits:** To keep the cognitive gears turning smoothly, engaging in activities that stimulate the brain is imperative. Whether it's the meditative strokes of adult colouring, the mental acrobatics of puzzles, the immersive world of hobbies, the enlightening pages of a good book, or the profound connection with nature, these pursuits actively contribute to the vitality of our mental faculties.

e) **Social Engagements:** The multifaceted impact of social interactions encompasses improved mental well-being, enhanced digestion through shared meals, the effervescence of happiness, boosted self-esteem, and the therapeutic presence of pets or the observation of animals in nature. Understanding the dynamics of the Law of Attraction in social relationships further deepens our comprehension of the interconnectedness of our mental well-being.

f) **Balancing Act:** Juggling the myriad facets of life requires a keen sense of balance and perspective. The contours of this equilibrium are subjective, varying from person to person.

g) **Mindfulness as a Skill:** Embracing mindfulness as a learned skill and integrating it into our lives provides a potent tool. It serves as a compass, directing us to the present moment and empowering us to navigate through intrusive thoughts about past events or future anxieties. While not universally effective, it stands as a valuable ally for many on their journey to emotional well-being.

Professional Support as a Stepping Stone: The acknowledgment that professional support might be necessary at times is a testament to the proactive stance we take toward self-care. Seeking help for emotional well-being is not a sign of weakness, but a courageous step toward nurturing one's mental health.

Self-awareness as a Sentinel: In the realm of emotional health, self-awareness emerges as a sentinel, a vigilant guardian against potential problems. By being attuned to our thoughts and emotions, we can intercept and address budding issues before they escalate into formidable challenges.

The Radiance of Self-Value and Respect: Recognizing our intrinsic worth and fostering self-respect lays the groundwork for positive mental health. Celebrating the seemingly modest, yet impactful contributions we make in the lives of others, fosters a sense of pride and fulfilment.

In the grand mosaic of our lives, it's paramount to appreciate our significance and the positive ripples we create, even in seemingly mundane actions that others hold dear. Let's ensure that, we not only recognize, but also take pride in the meaningful contributions we make.

The Art of Now: Colouring Your Way to Mindfulness

'The soul becomes dyed with the color of its thoughts'
Marcus Aurelius[105]

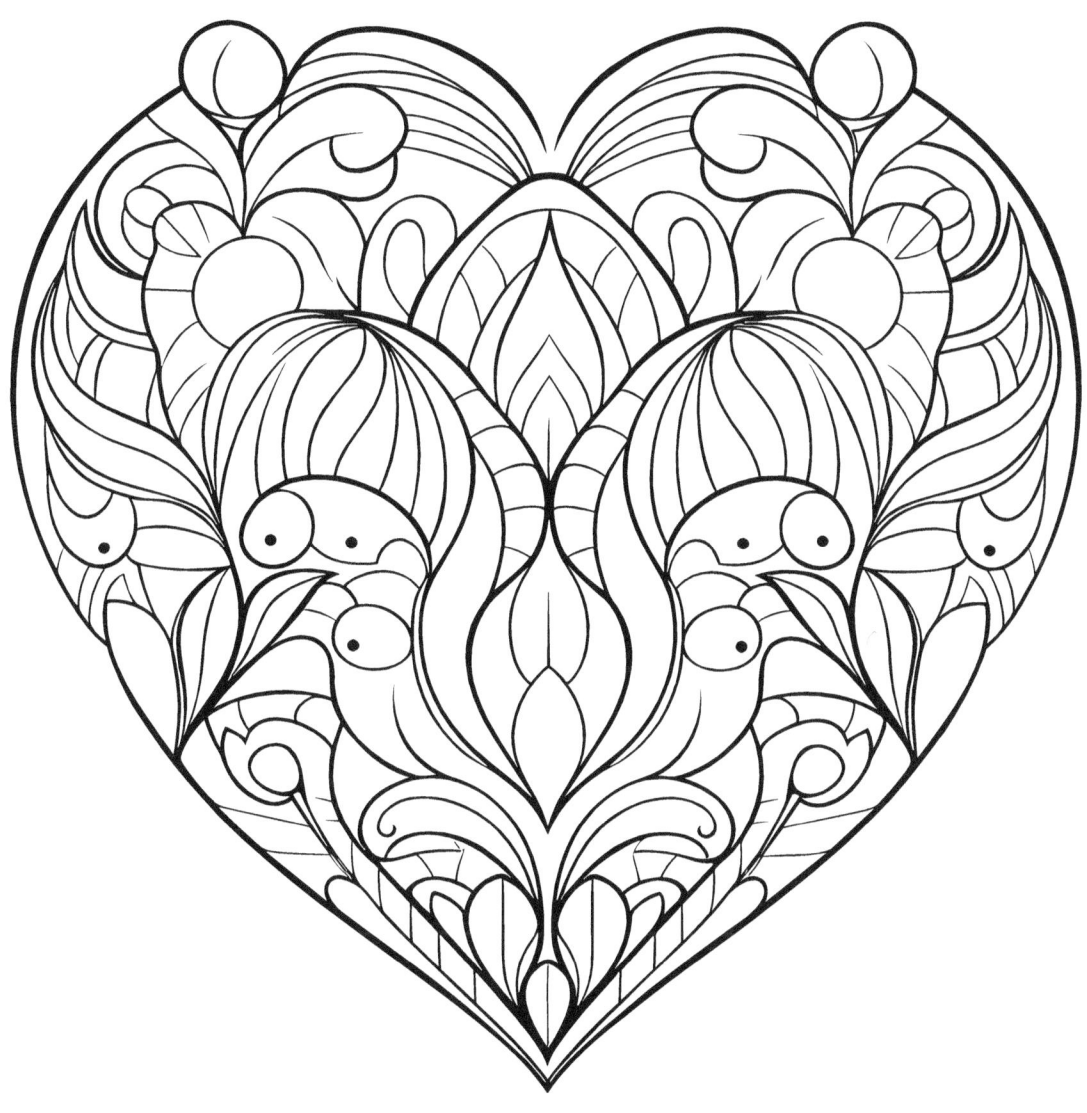

---
[105]'Marcus Aurelius', Marcus Aurelius Quotes (Web Page) < https://www.brainyquote.com/quotes/marcus_aurelius_131341 >.

Joe Aguilus

*Blank by
Design*

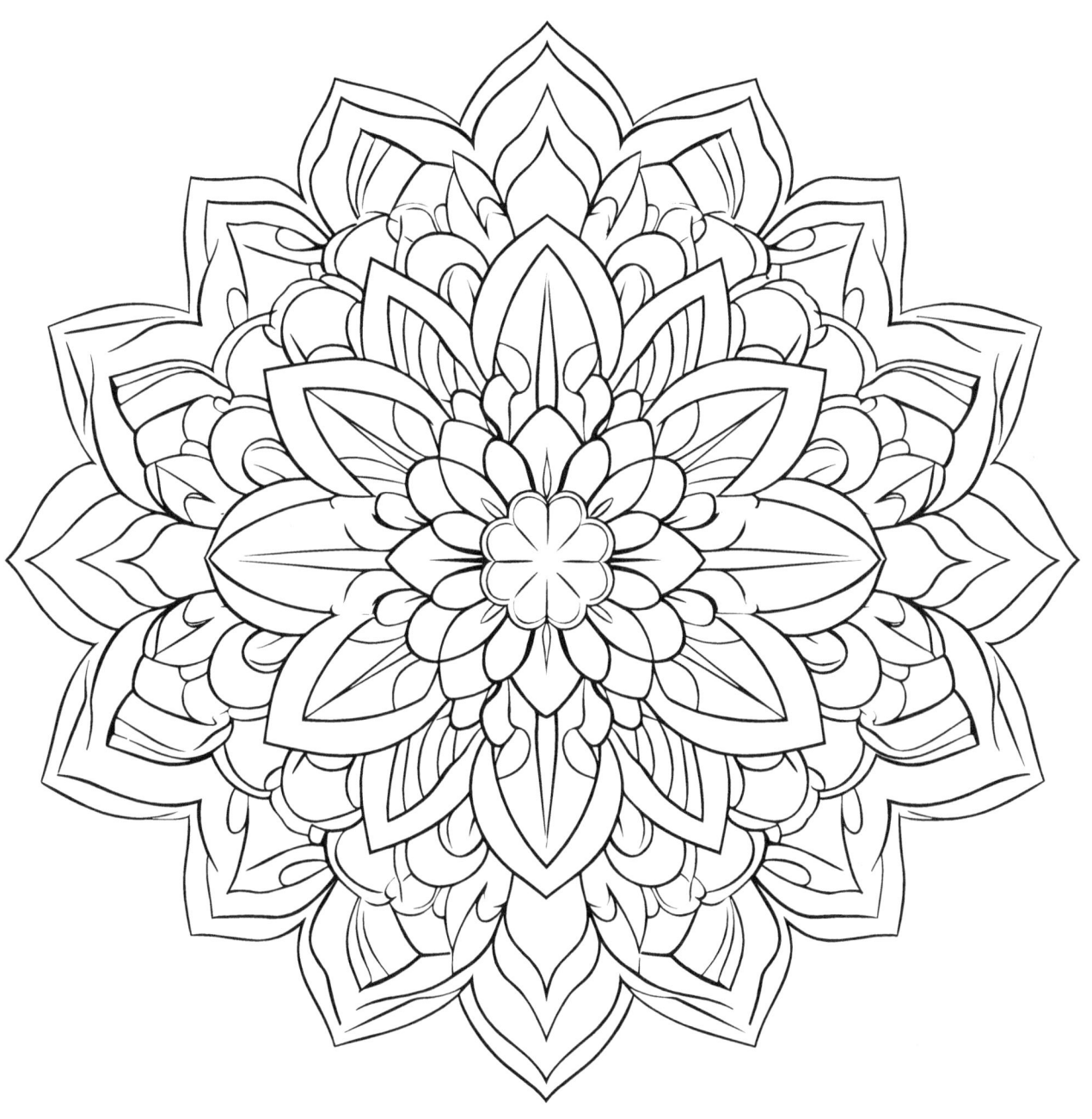

Blank by Design

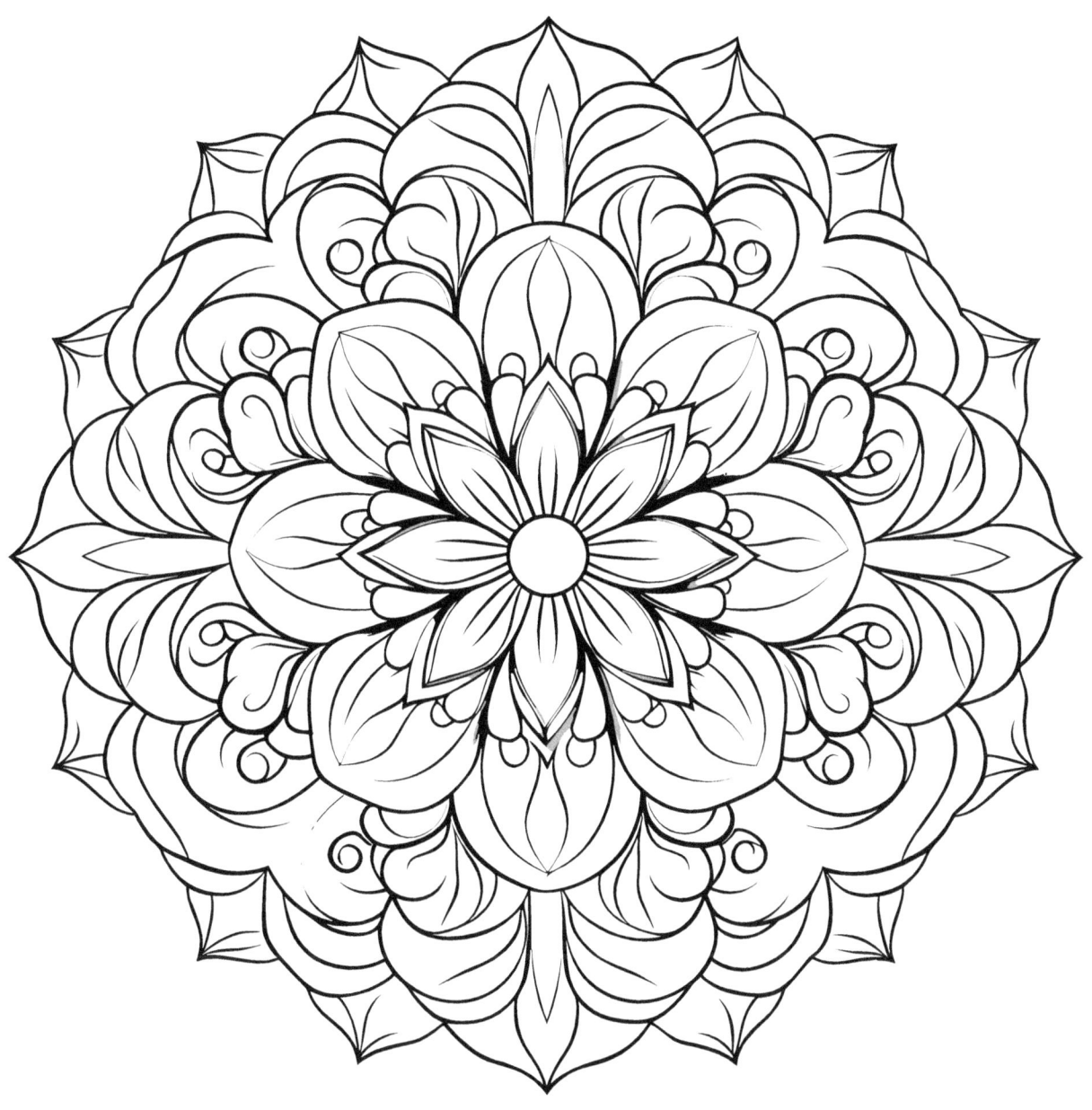

Blank by Design

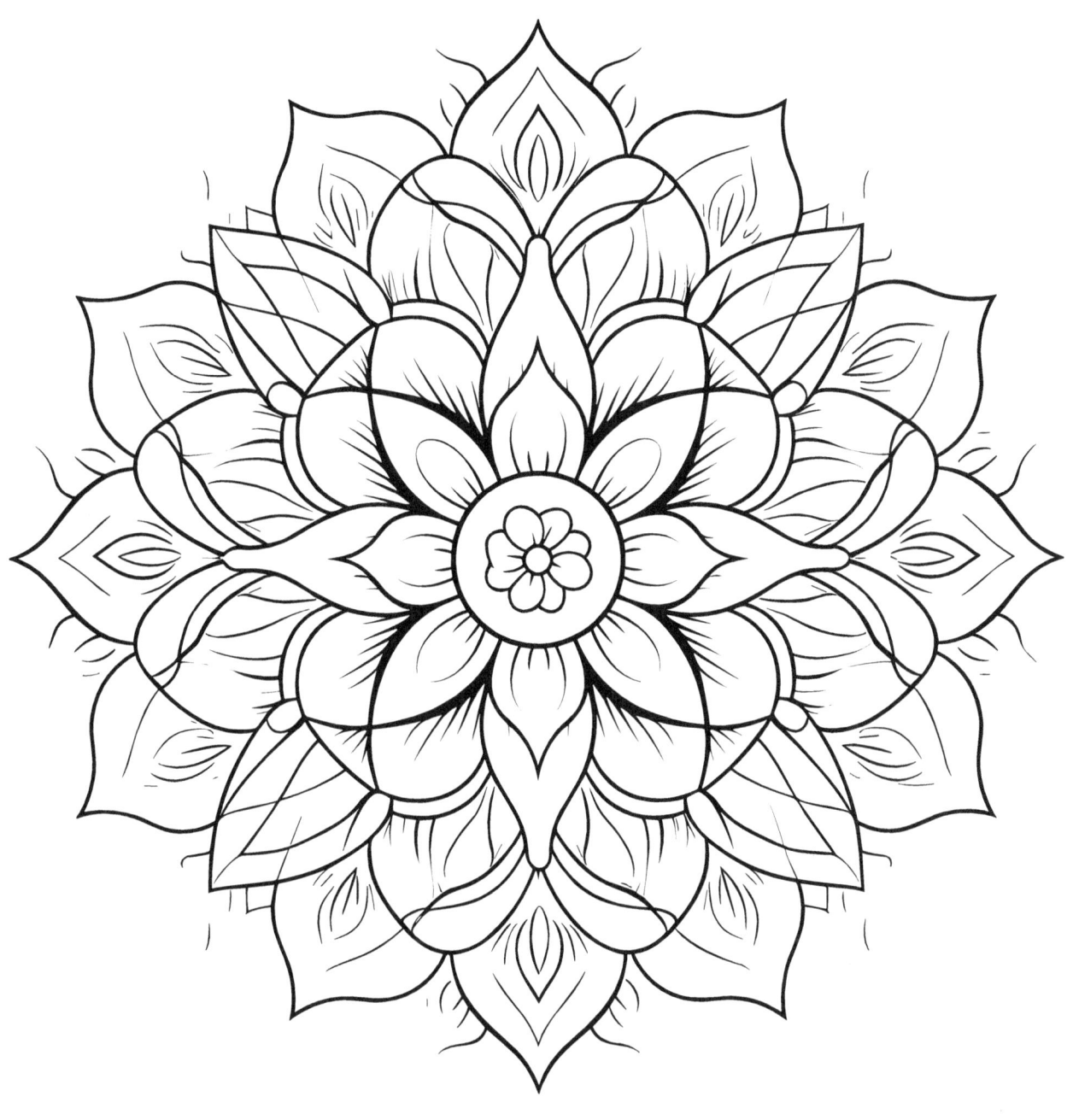

Blank by Design

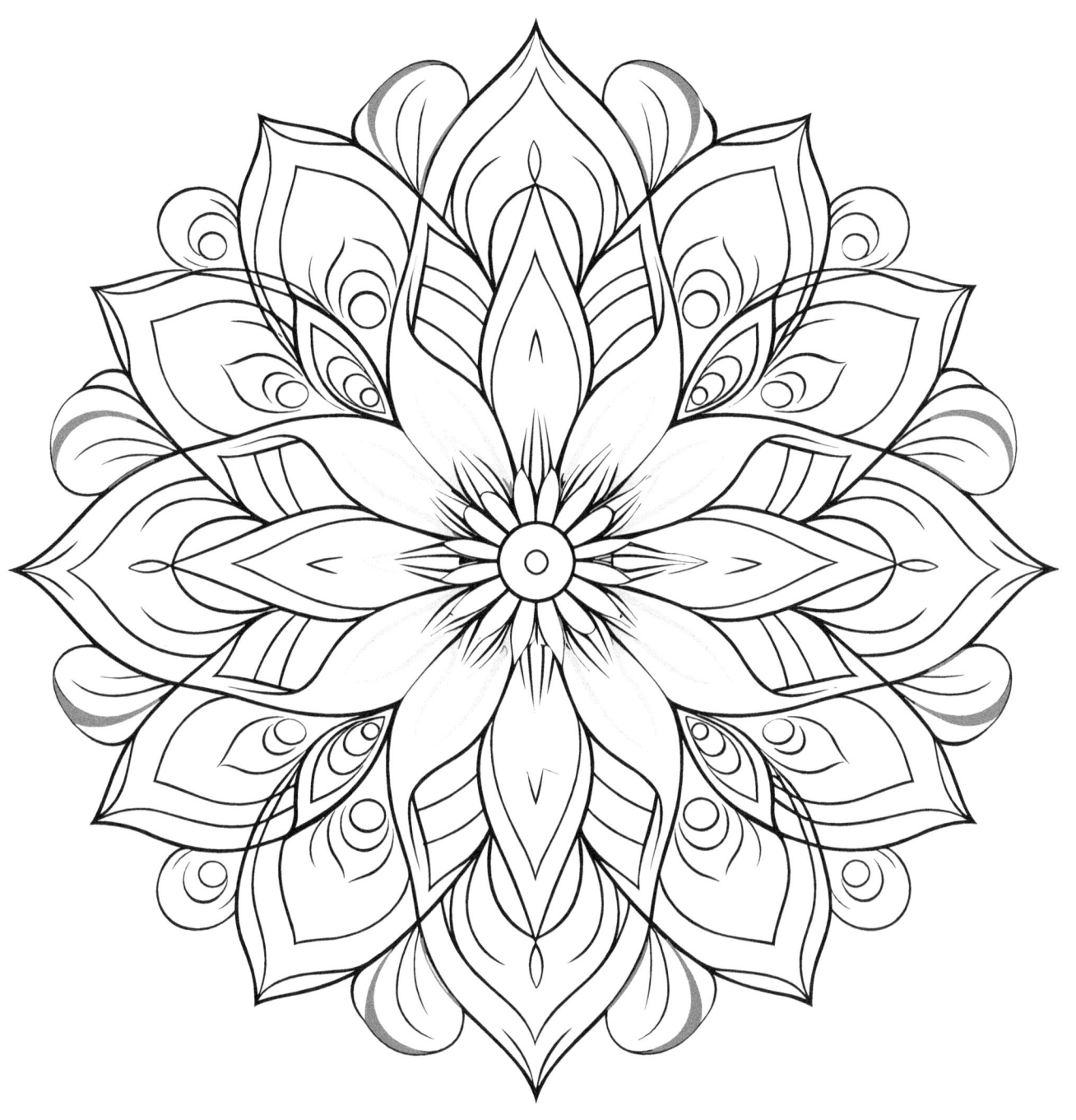

Blank by Design

Balanced Mind Balanced Life

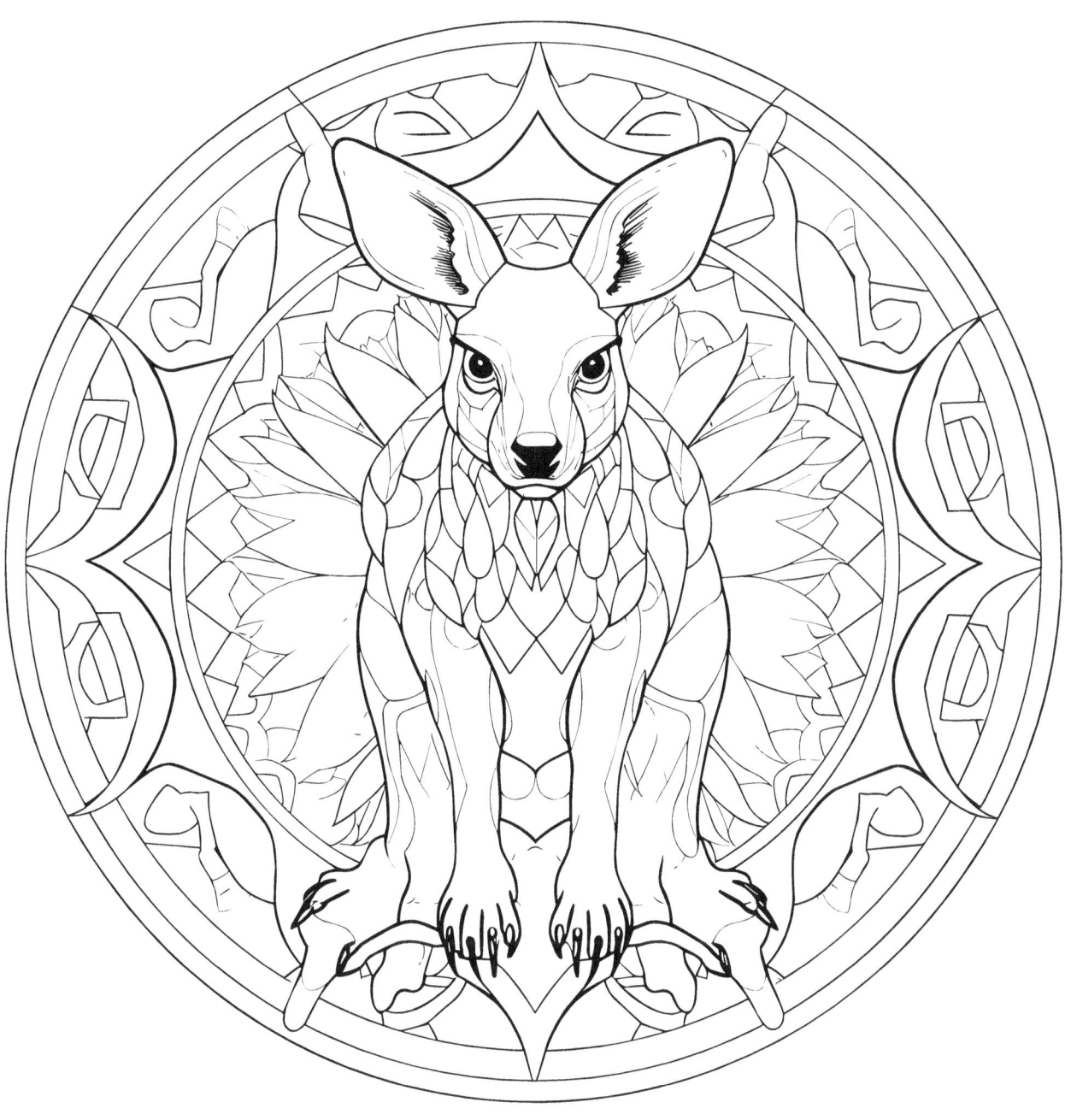

Blank by Design

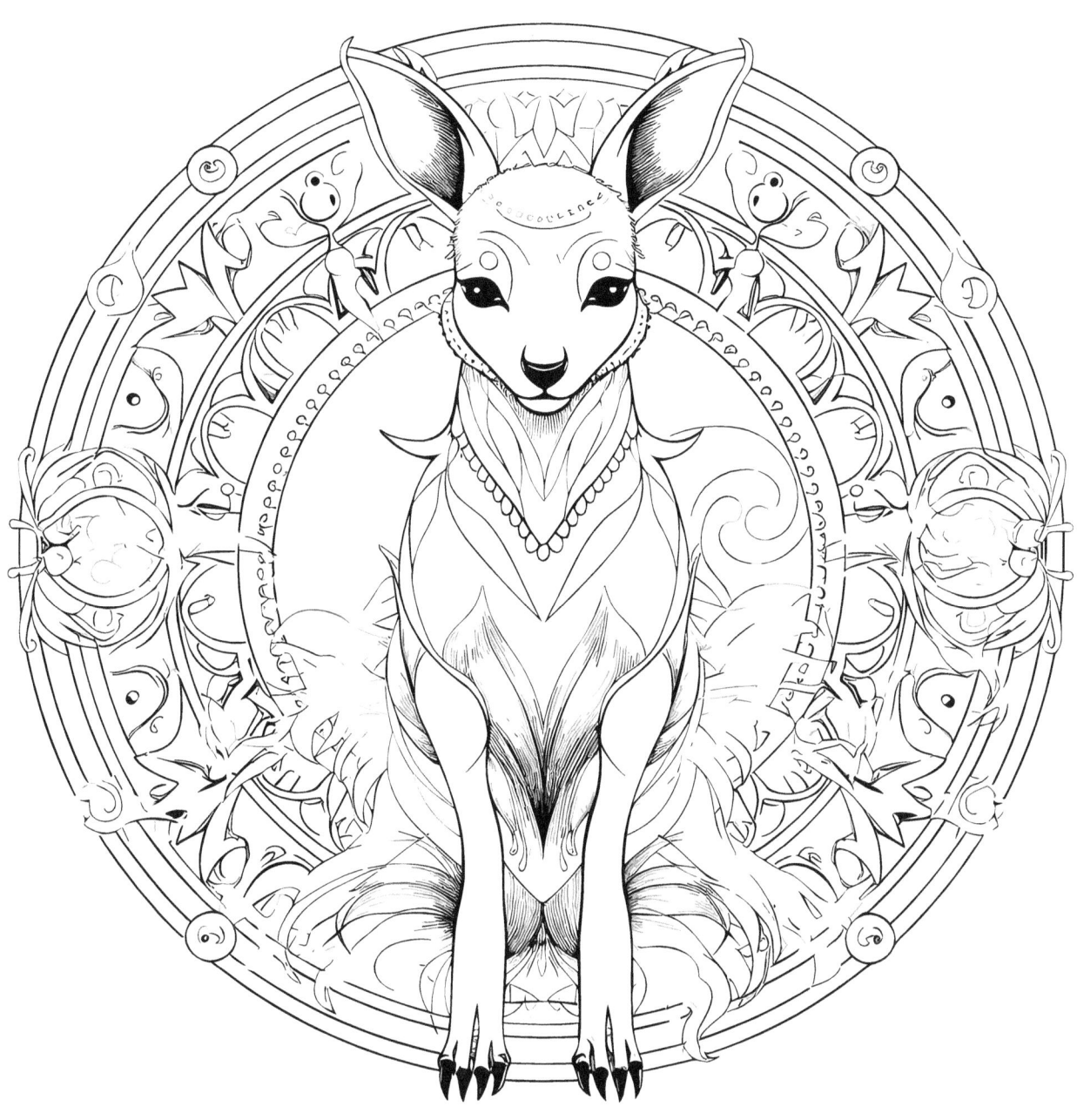

Blank by Design

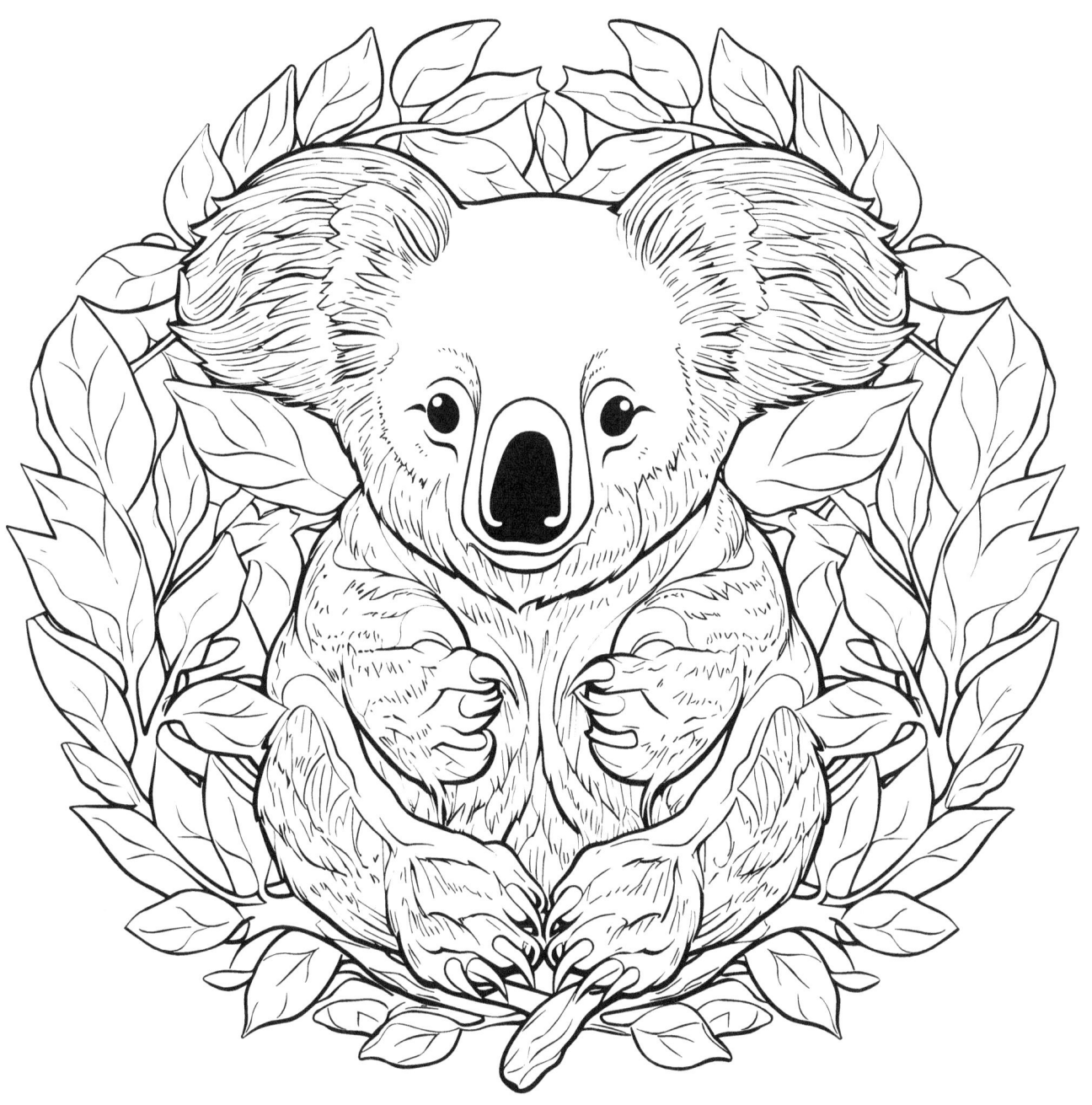

Blank by Design

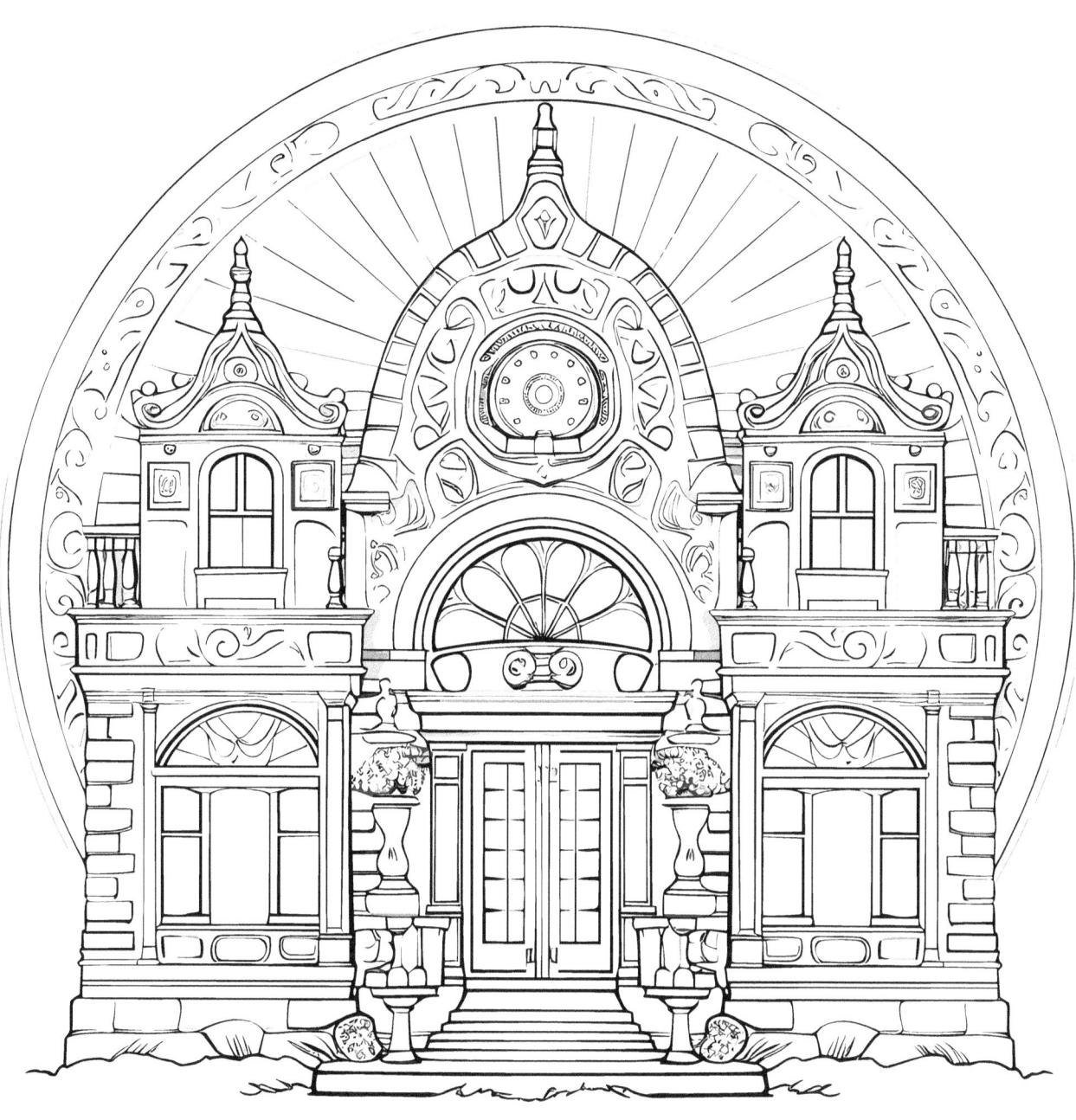

Blank by Design

Balanced Mind Balanced Life

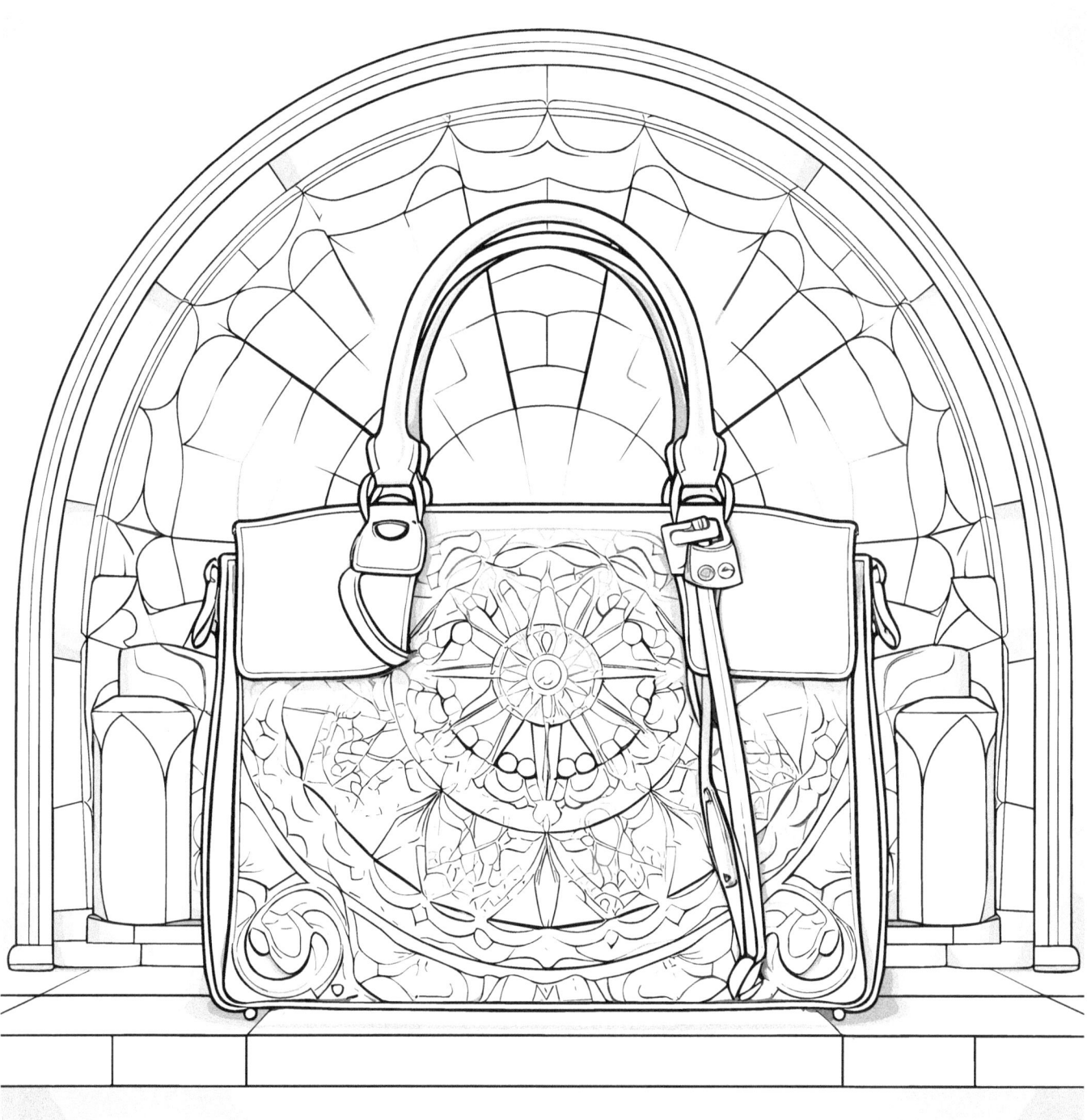

Blank by Design

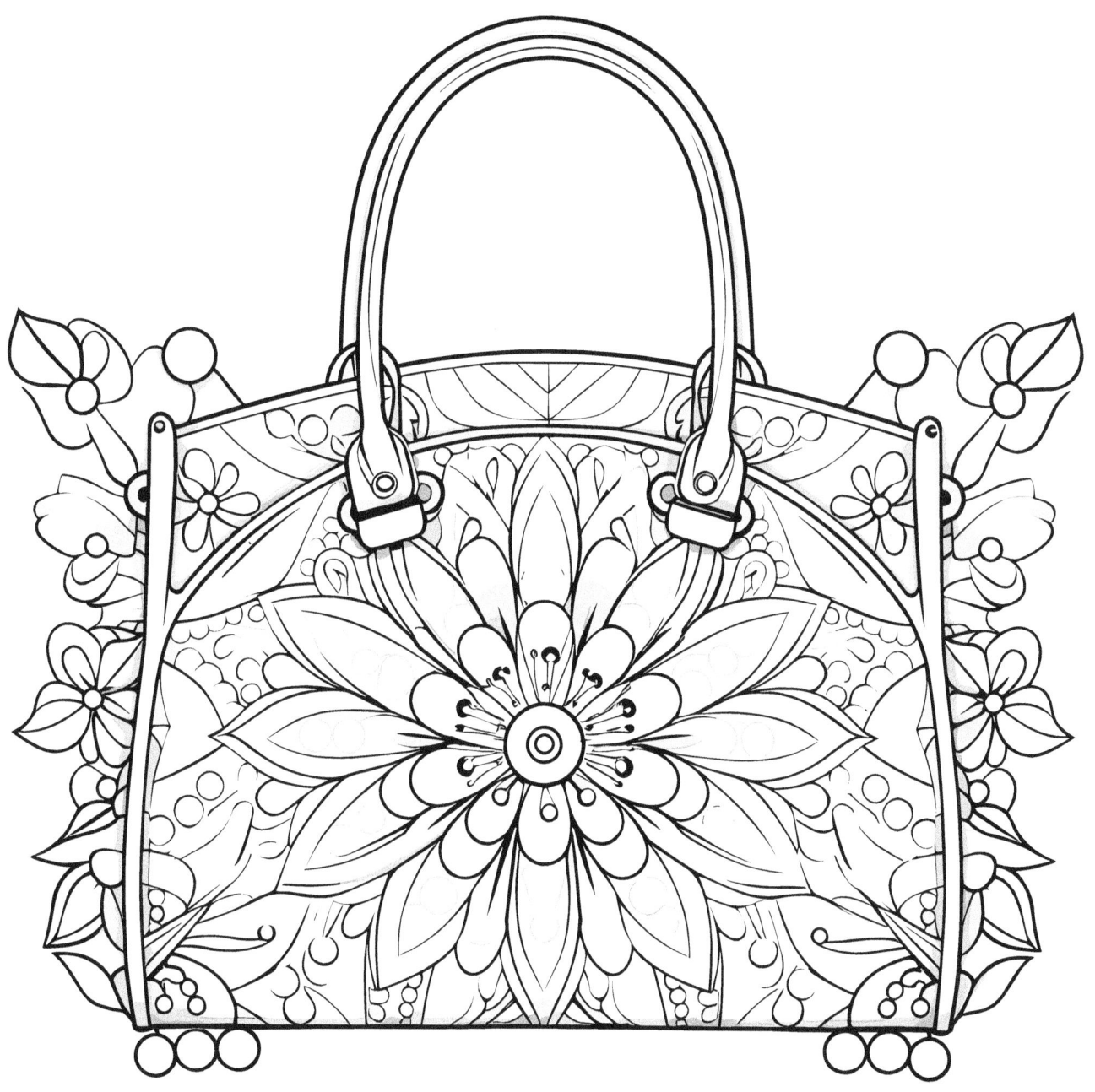

Blank by Design

Balanced Mind Balanced Life

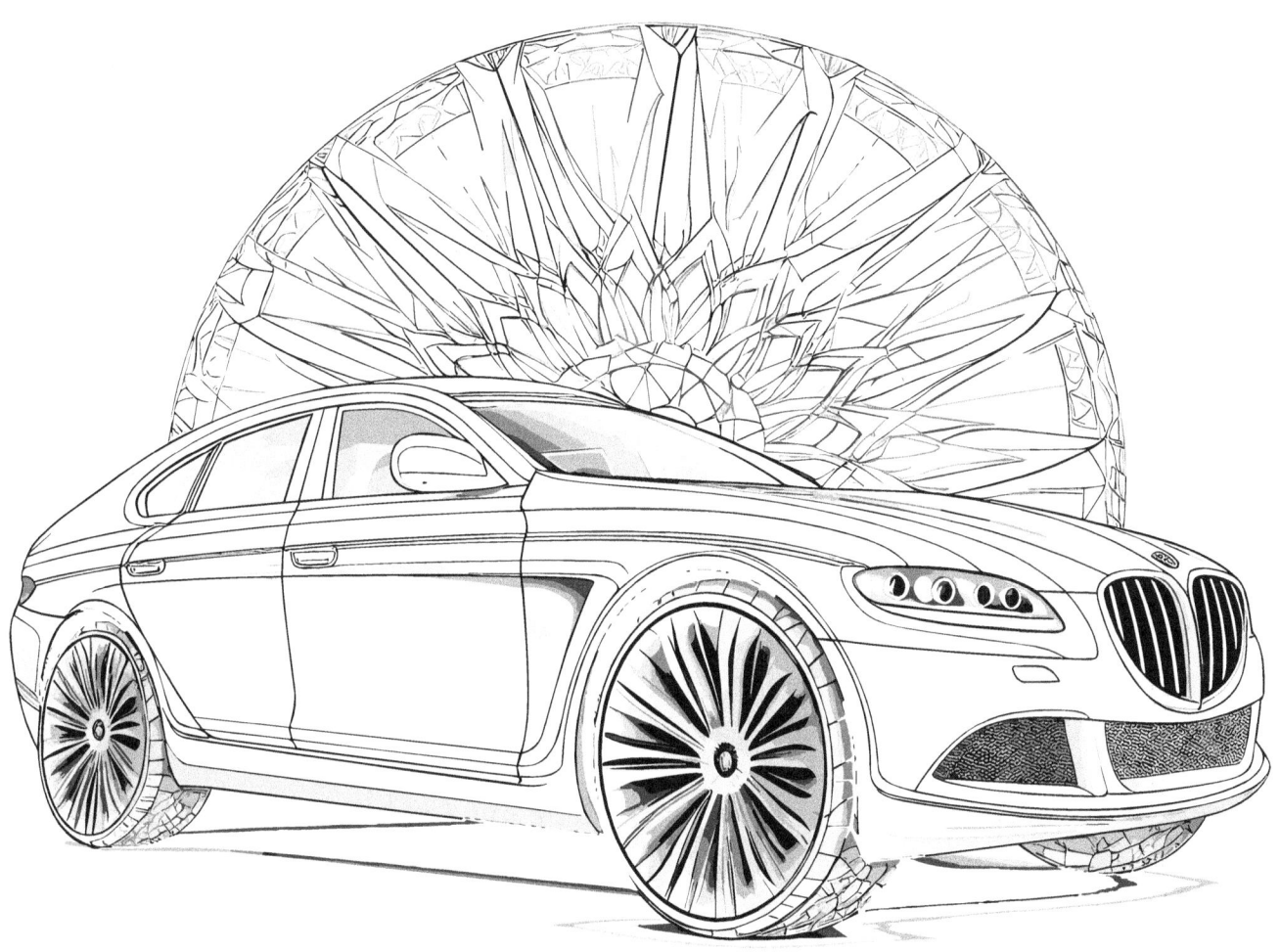

Blank by Design

Balanced Mind Balanced Life

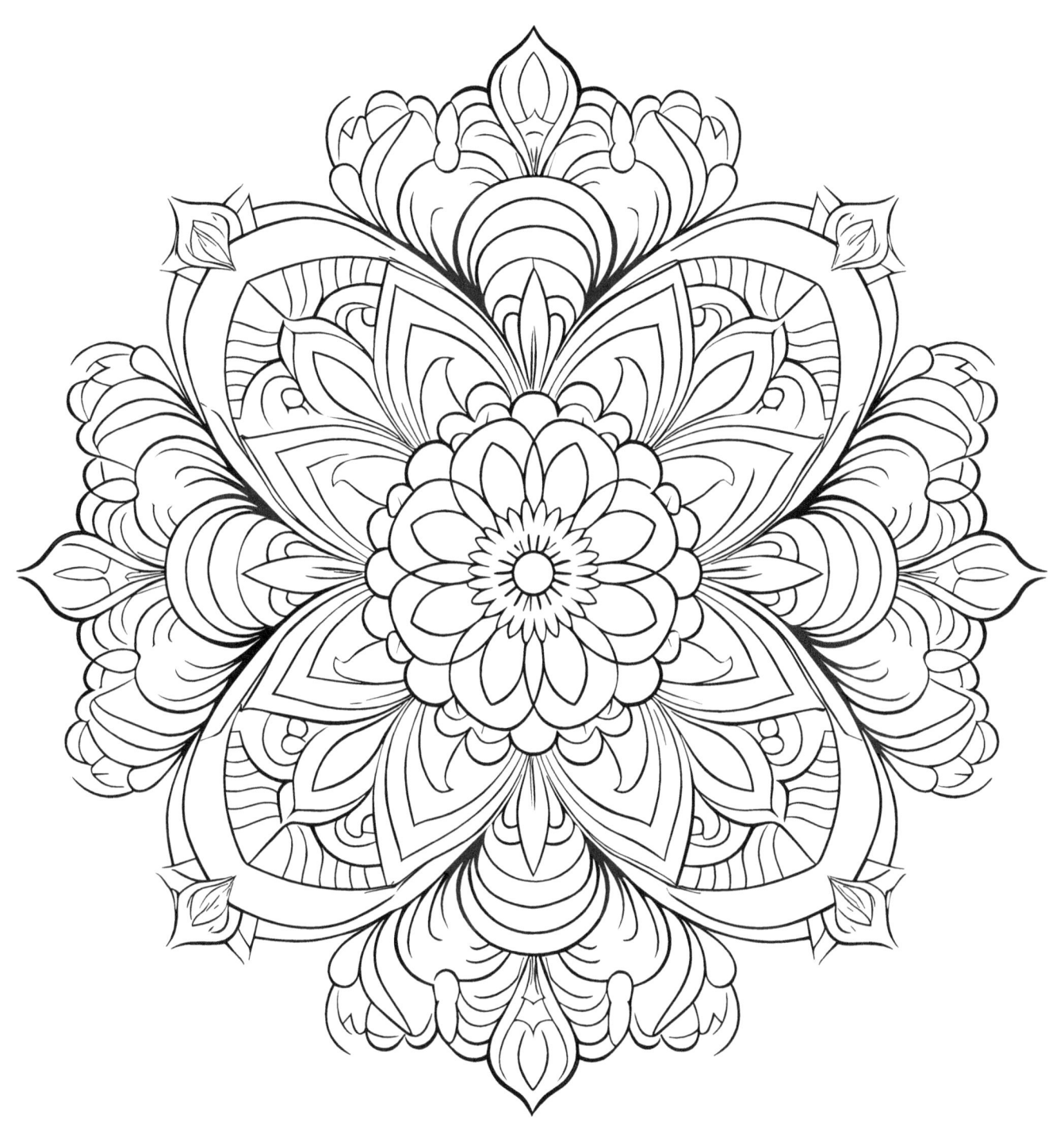

Blank by Design

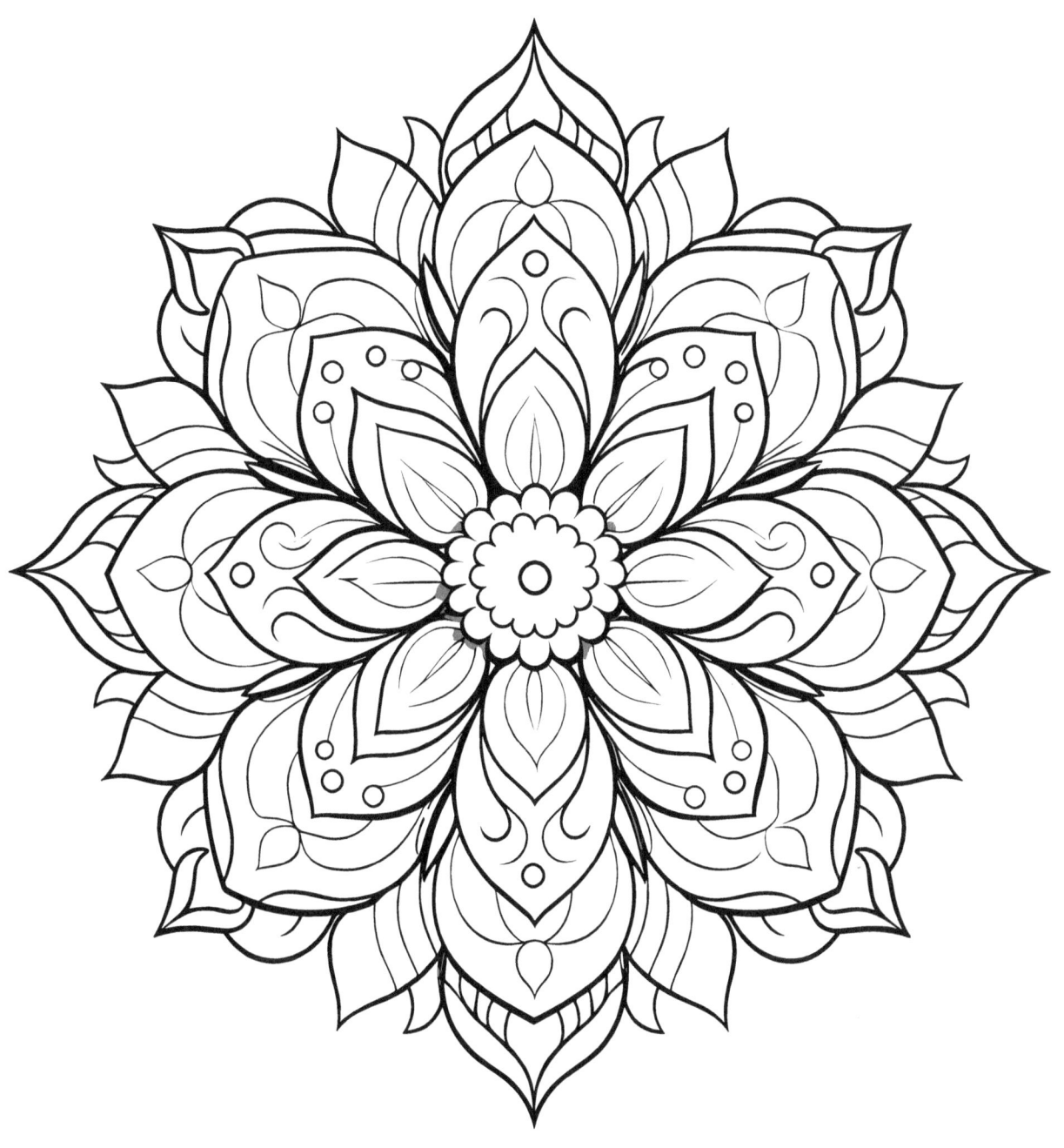

Blank by Design

Balanced Mind Balanced Life

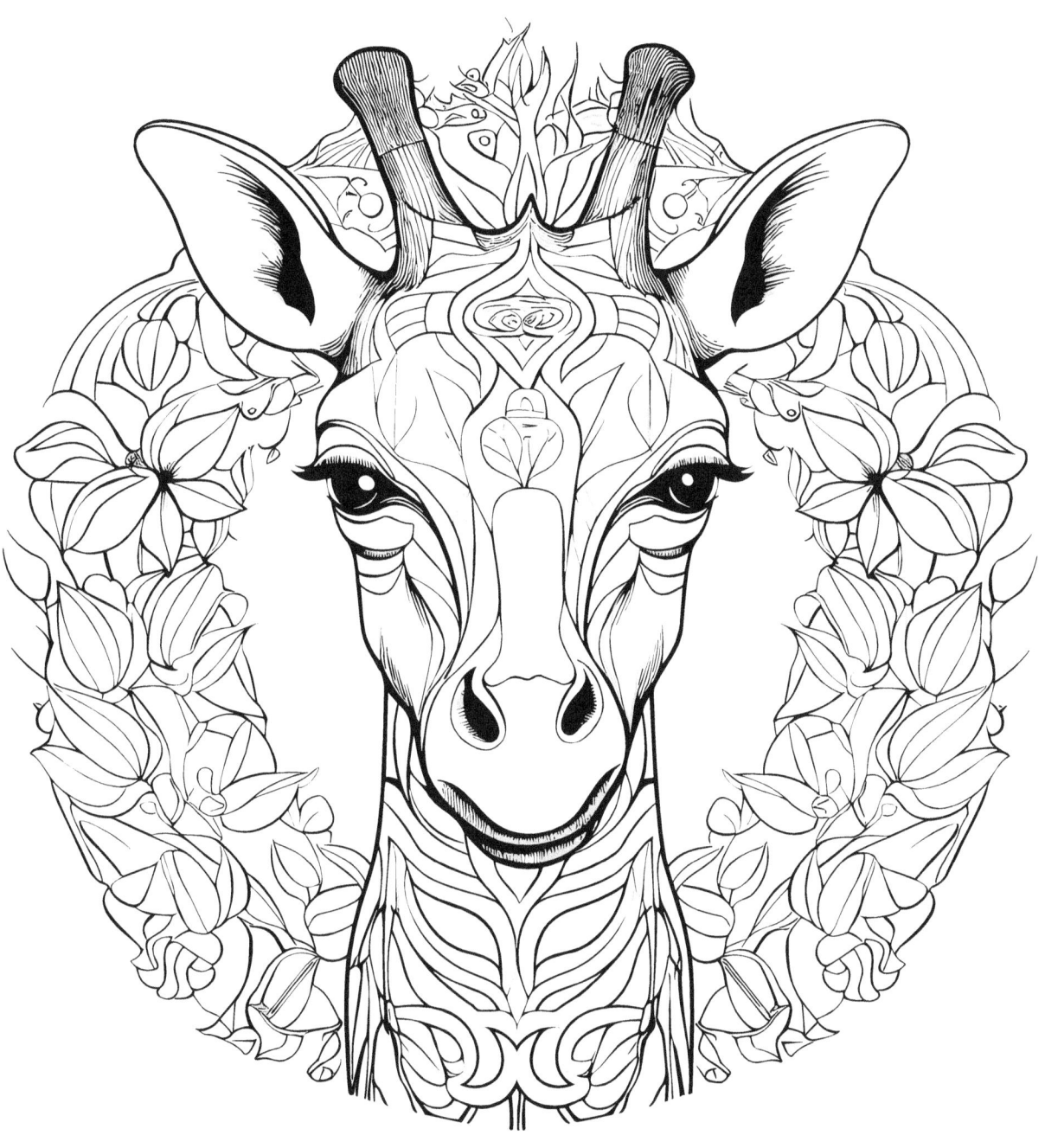

Blank by Design

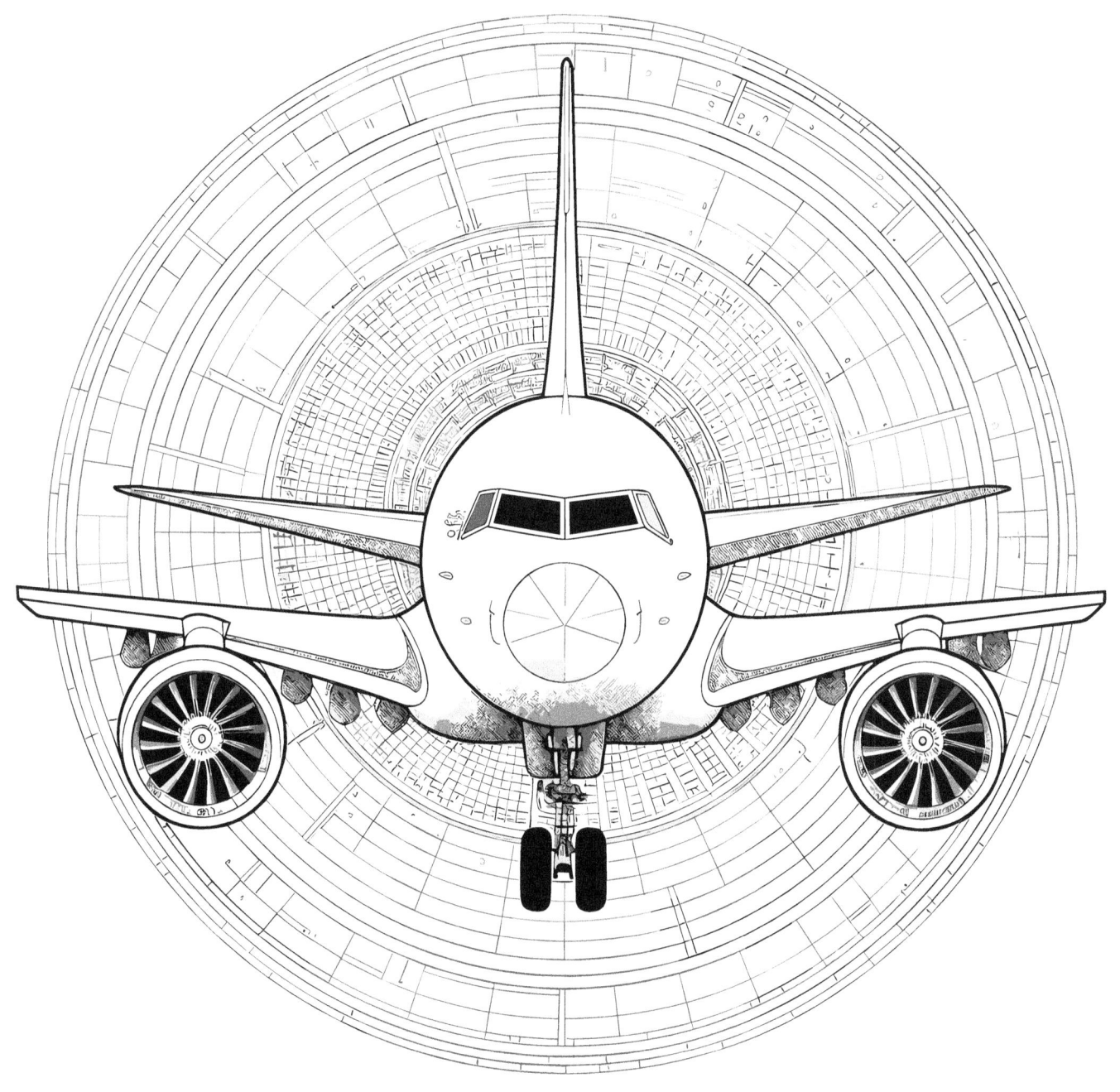

Blank by Design

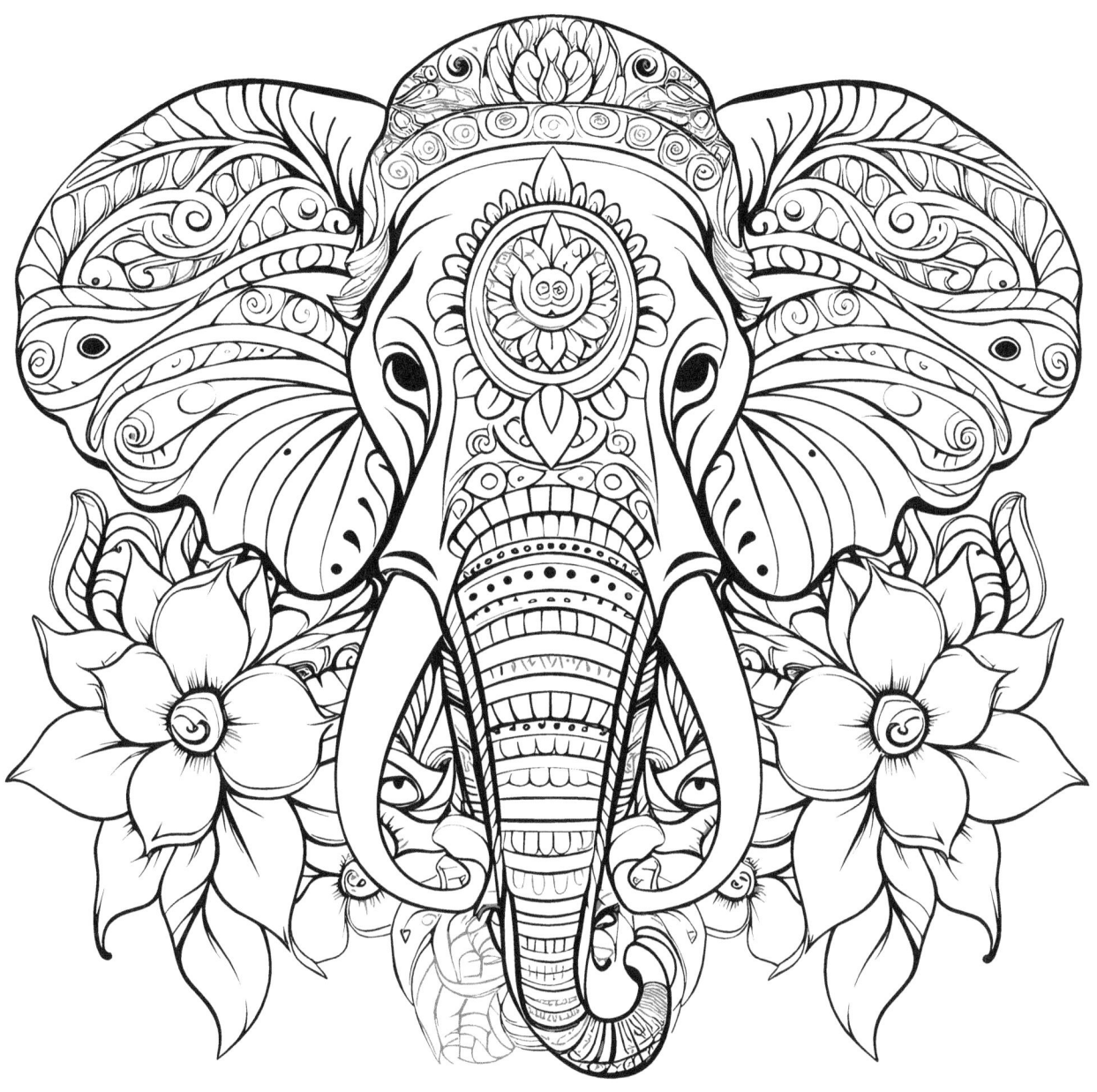

Blank by Design

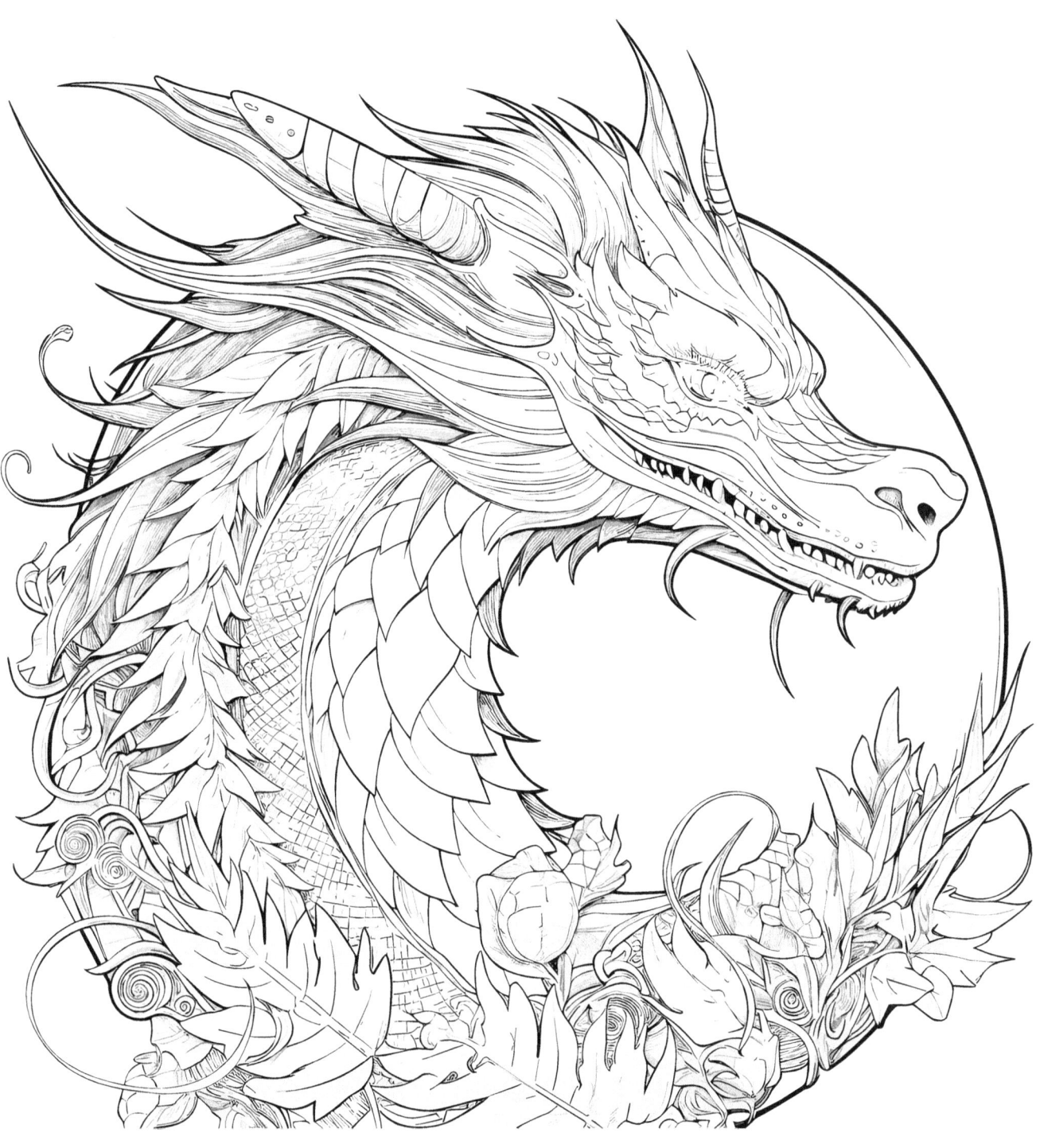

Blank by Design

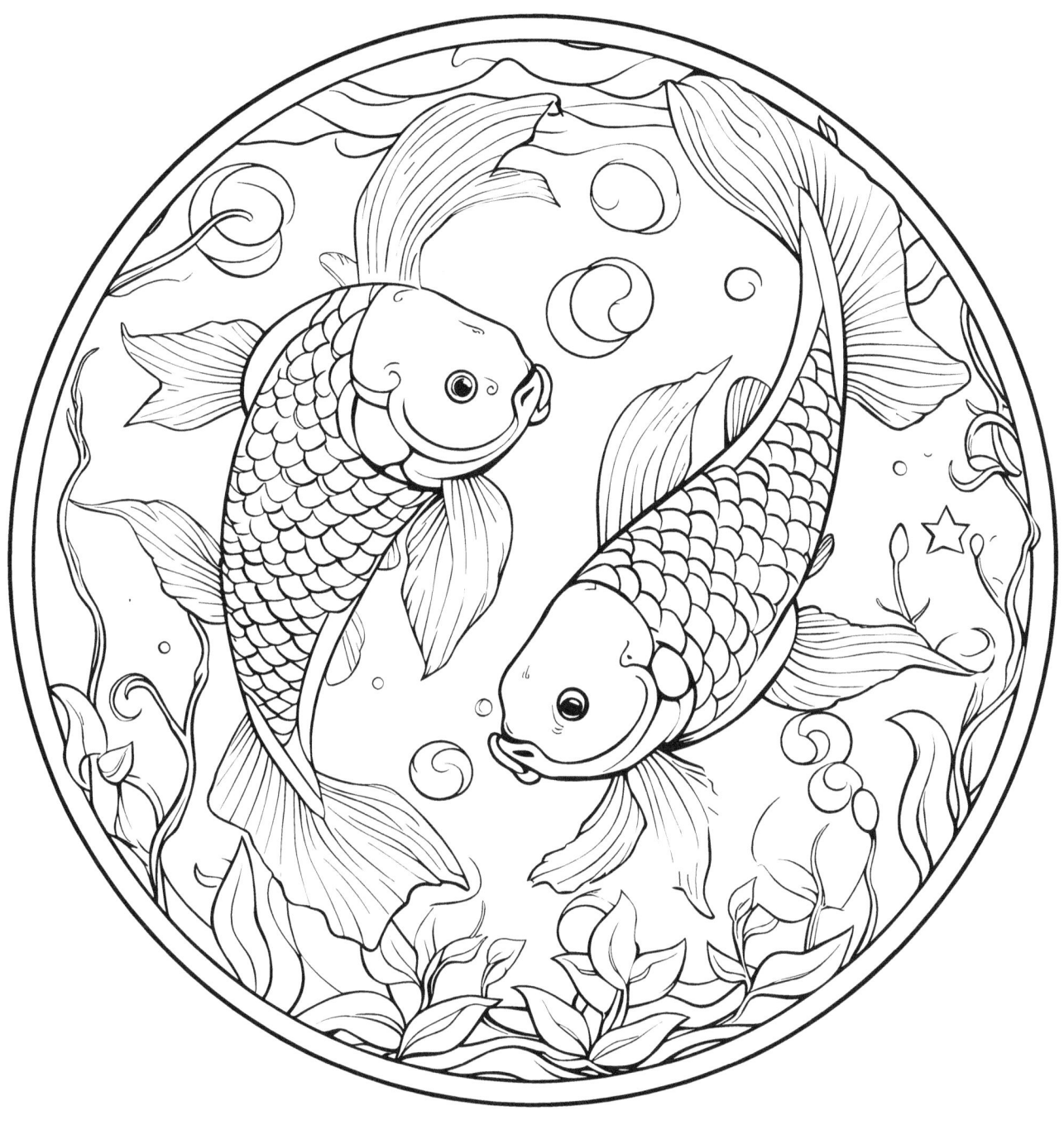

Joe Aguilus

Blank by Design

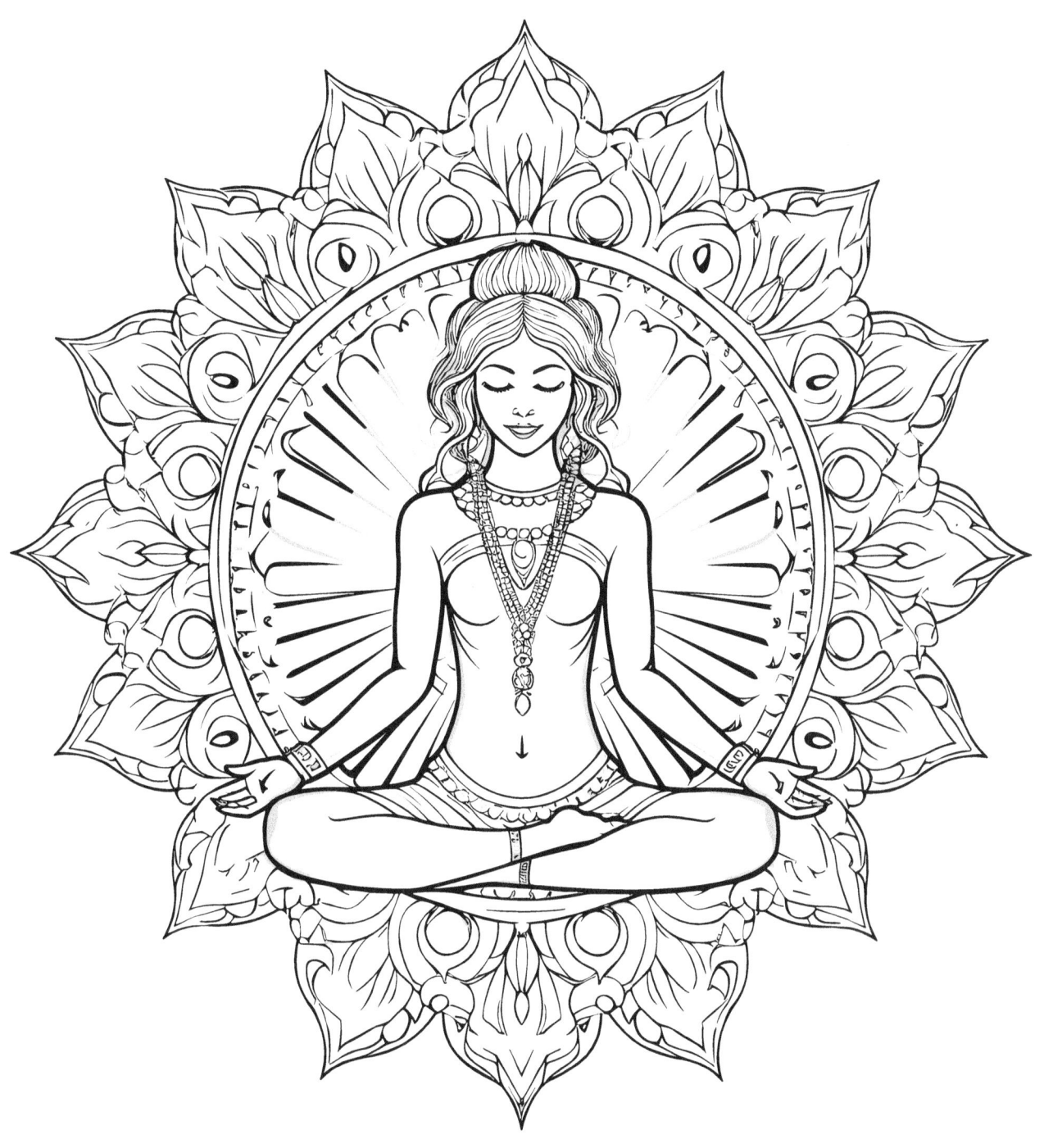

Blank by Design

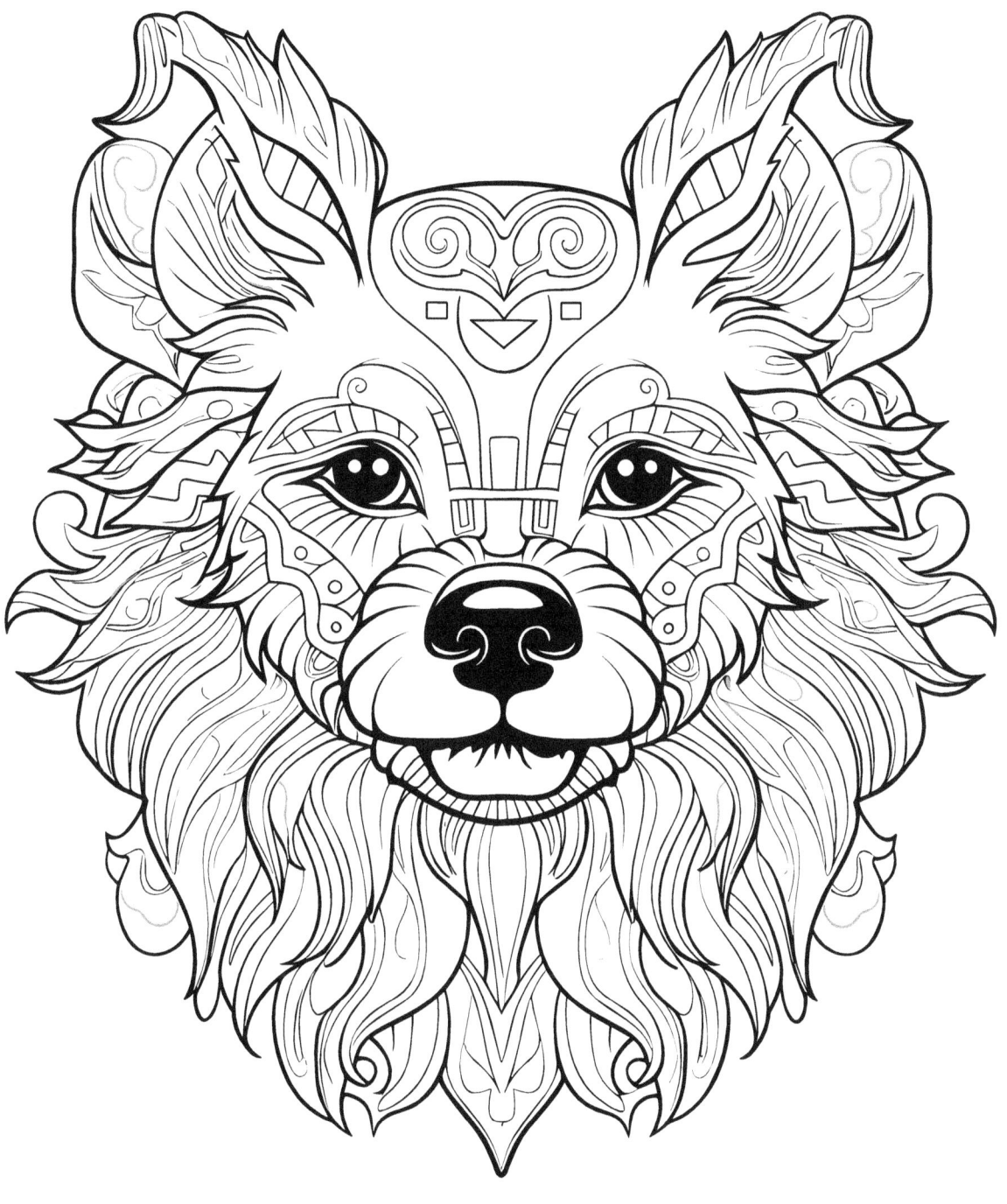

Blank by Design

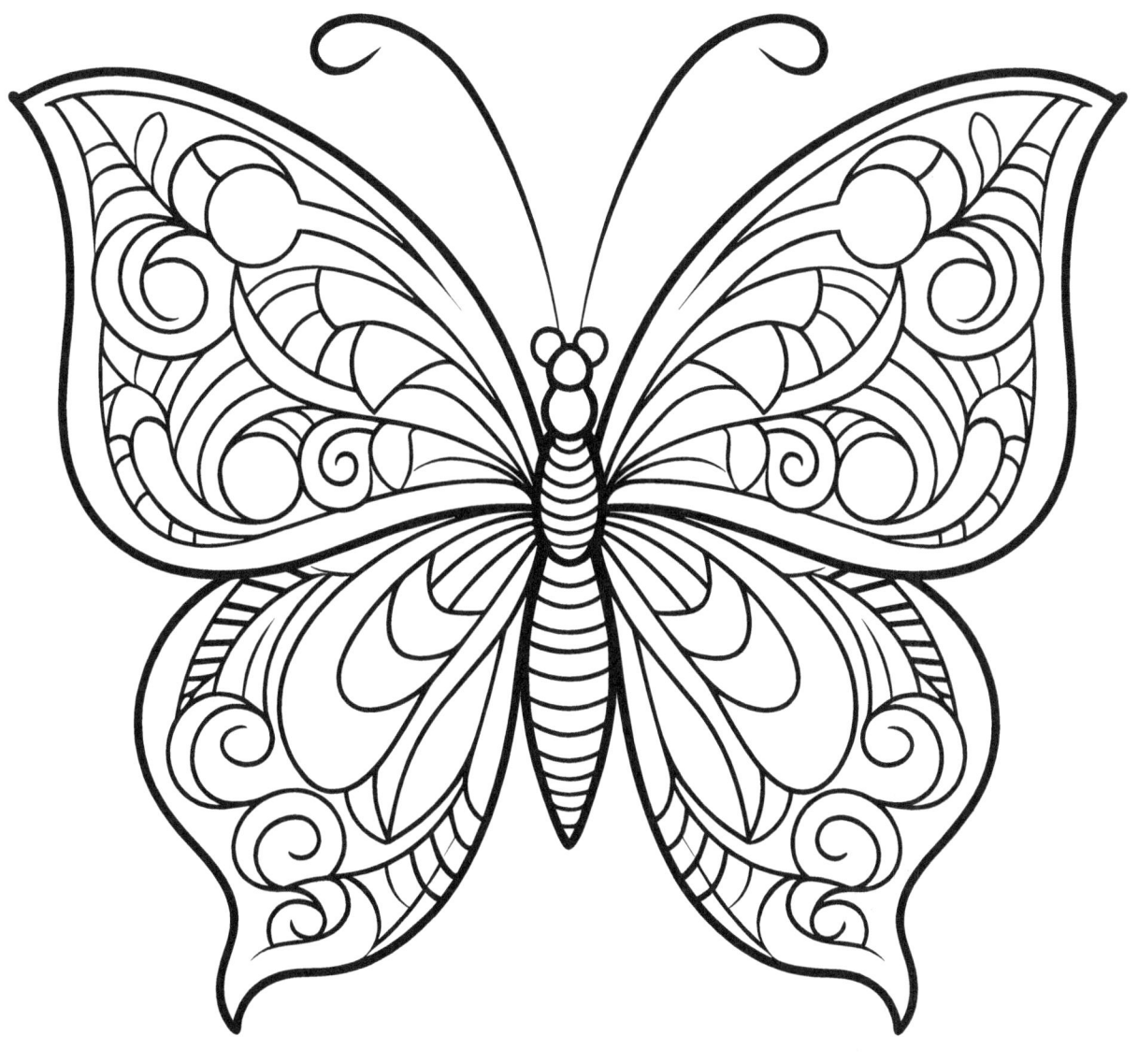

Blank by Design

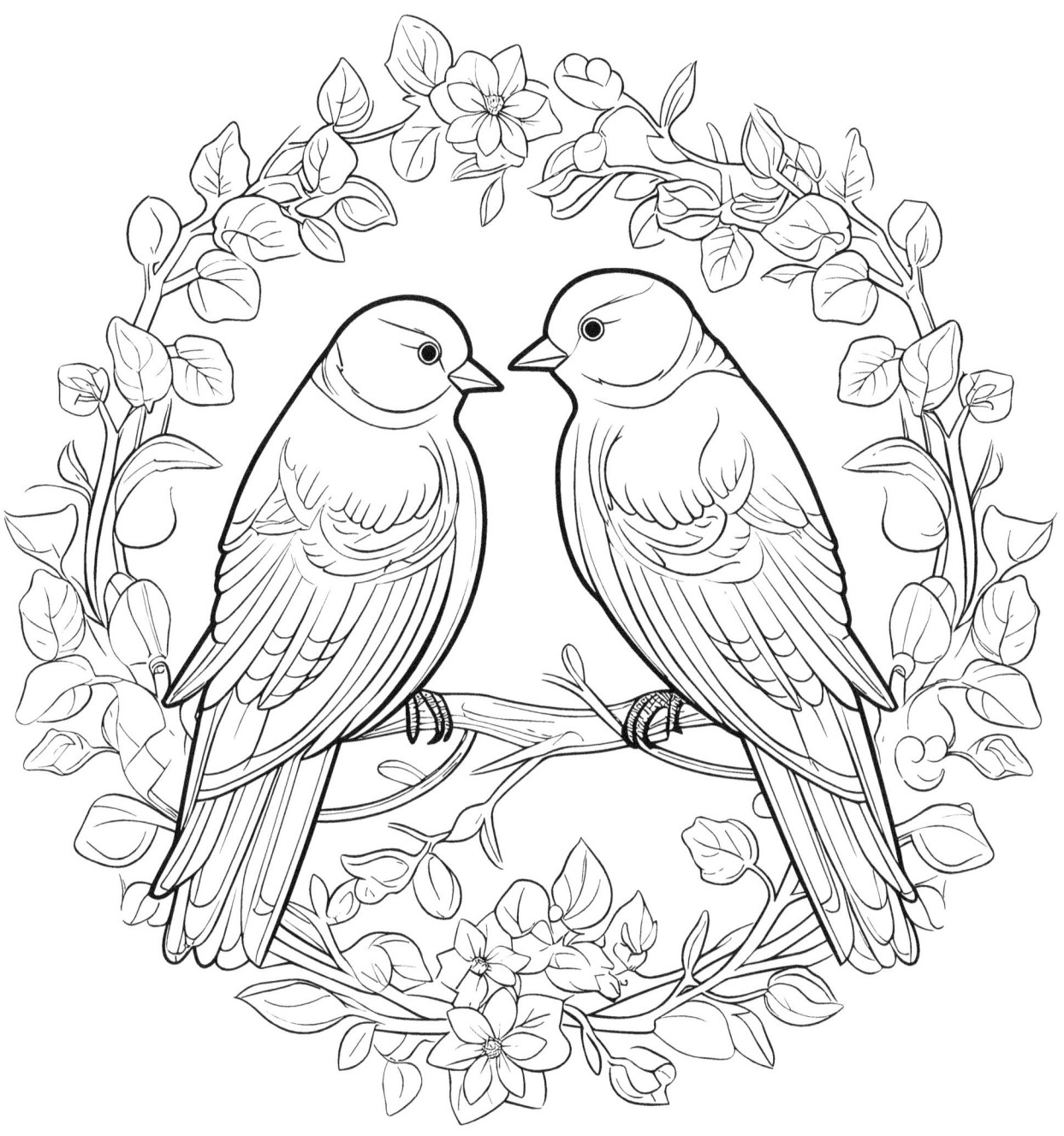

Blank by Design

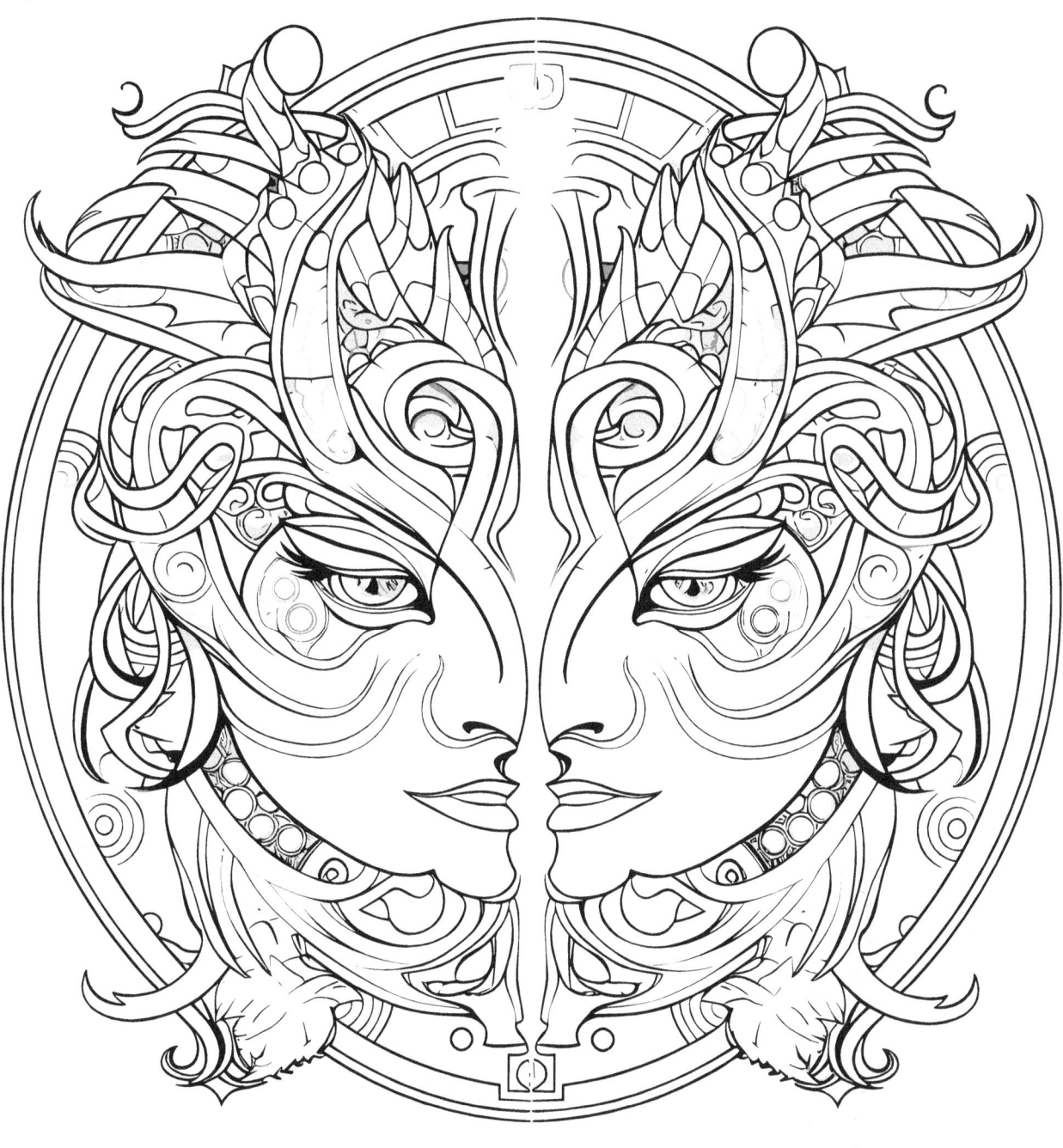

Blank by Design

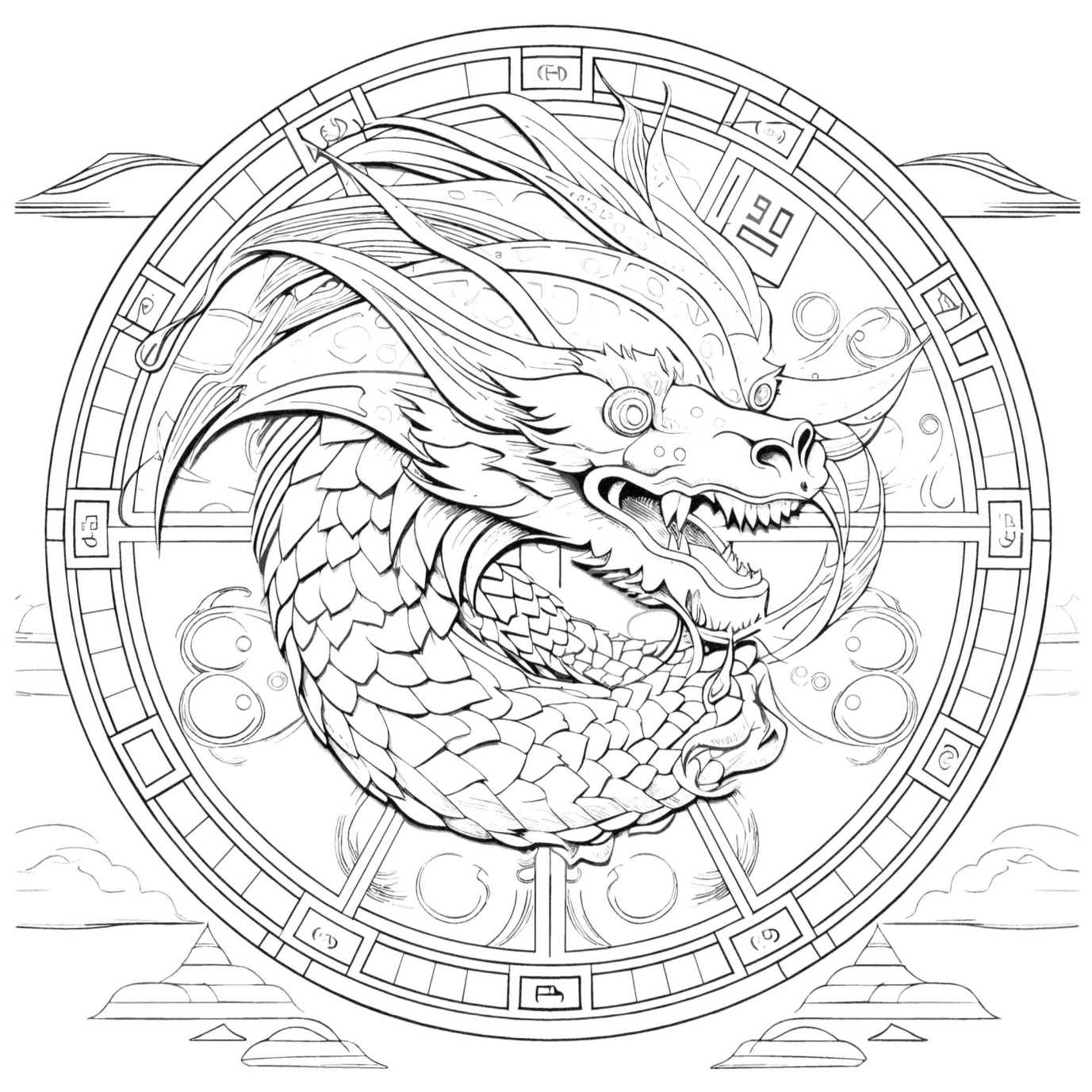

Blank by Design

Balanced Mind Balanced Life

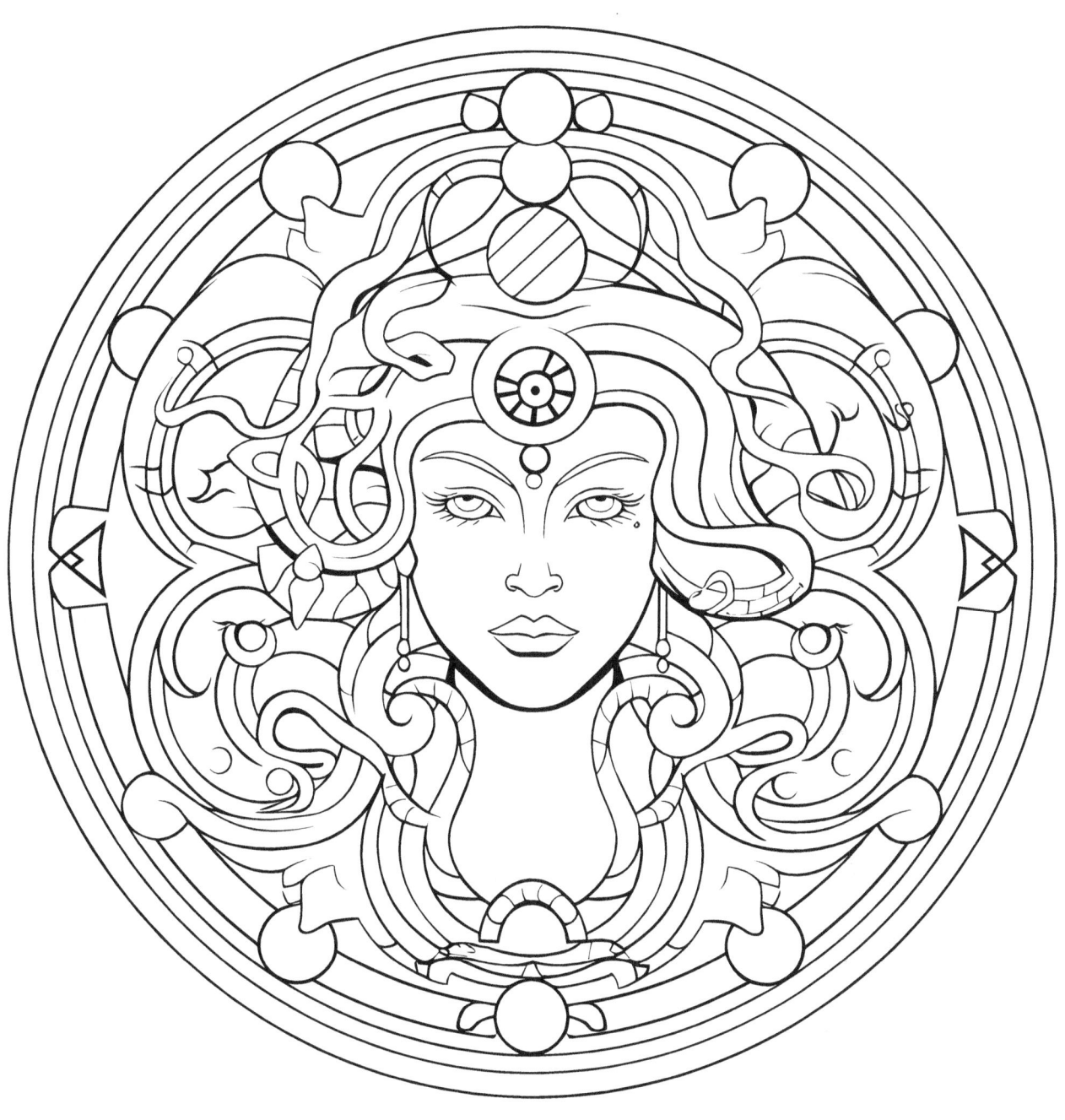

Blank by Design

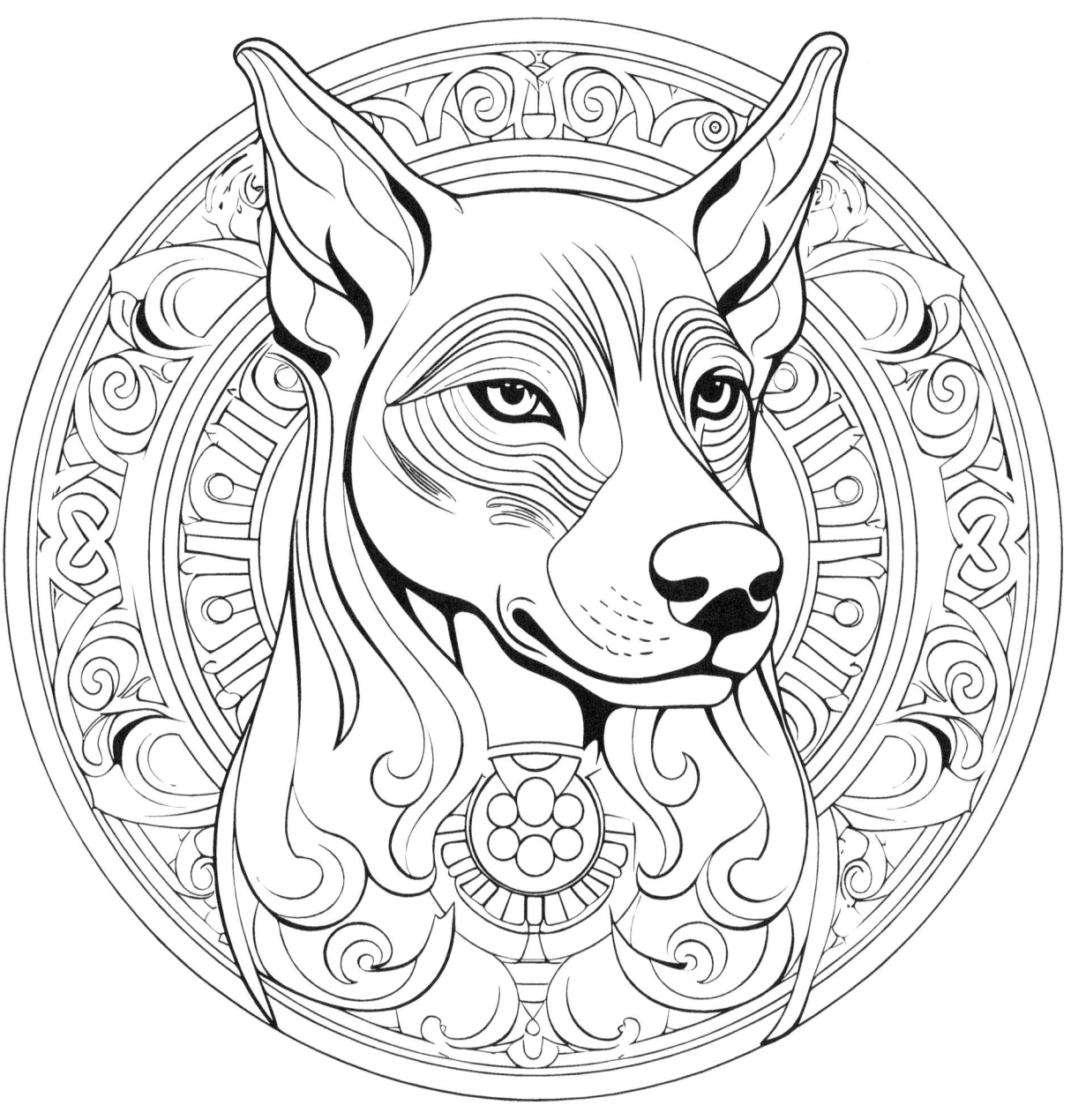

Blank by Design

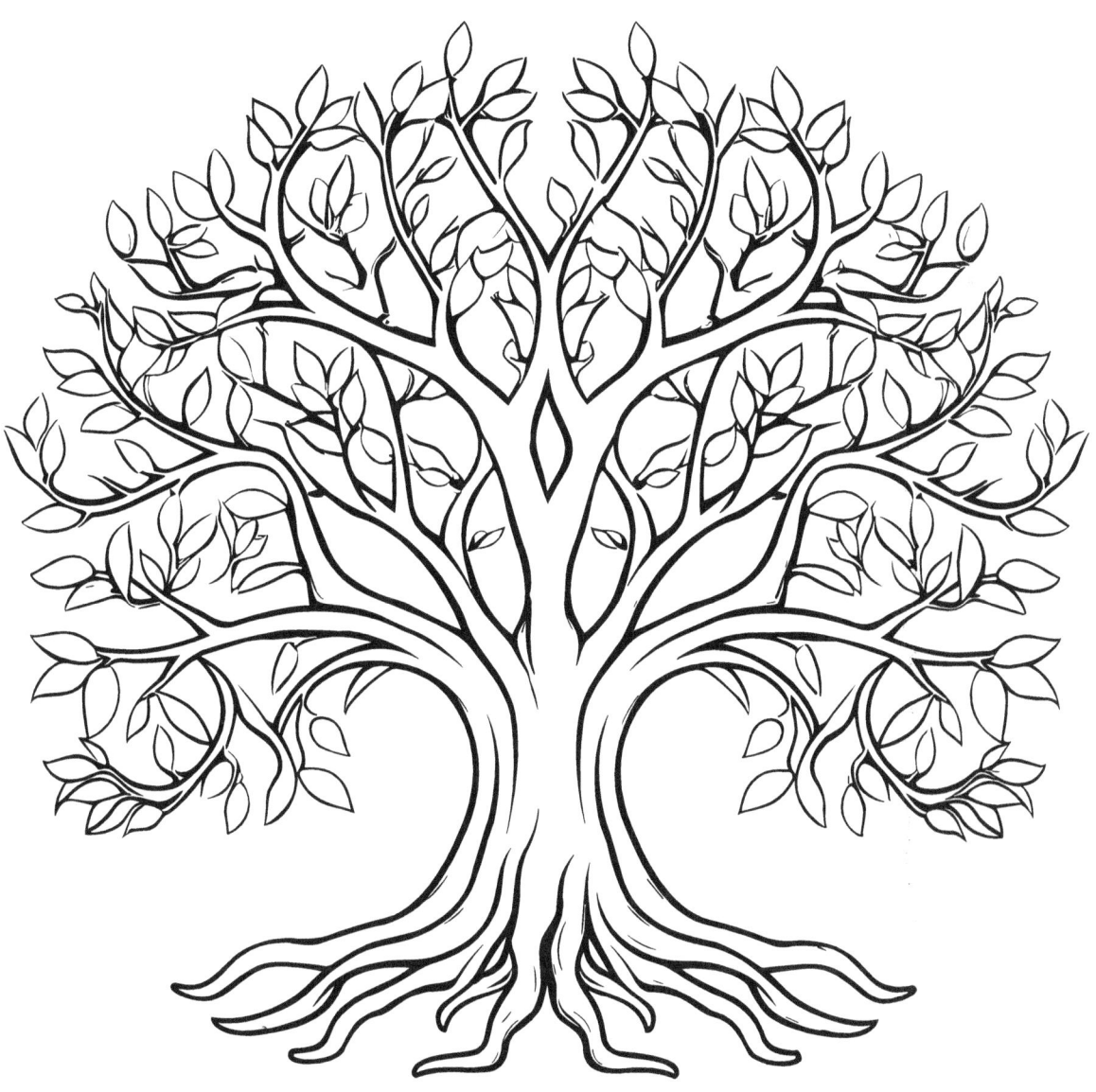

Blank by Design

Balanced Mind Balanced Life

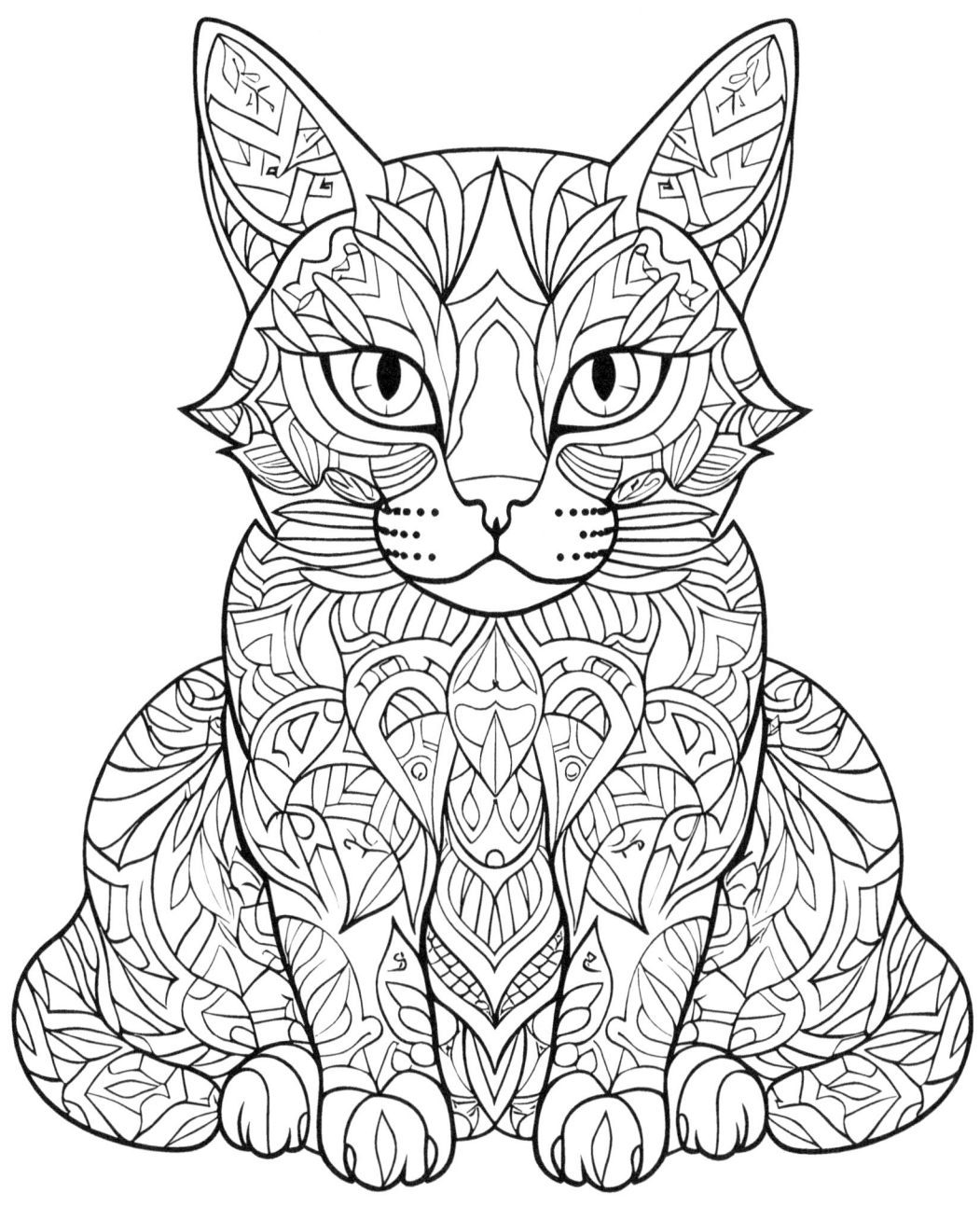

Blank by Design

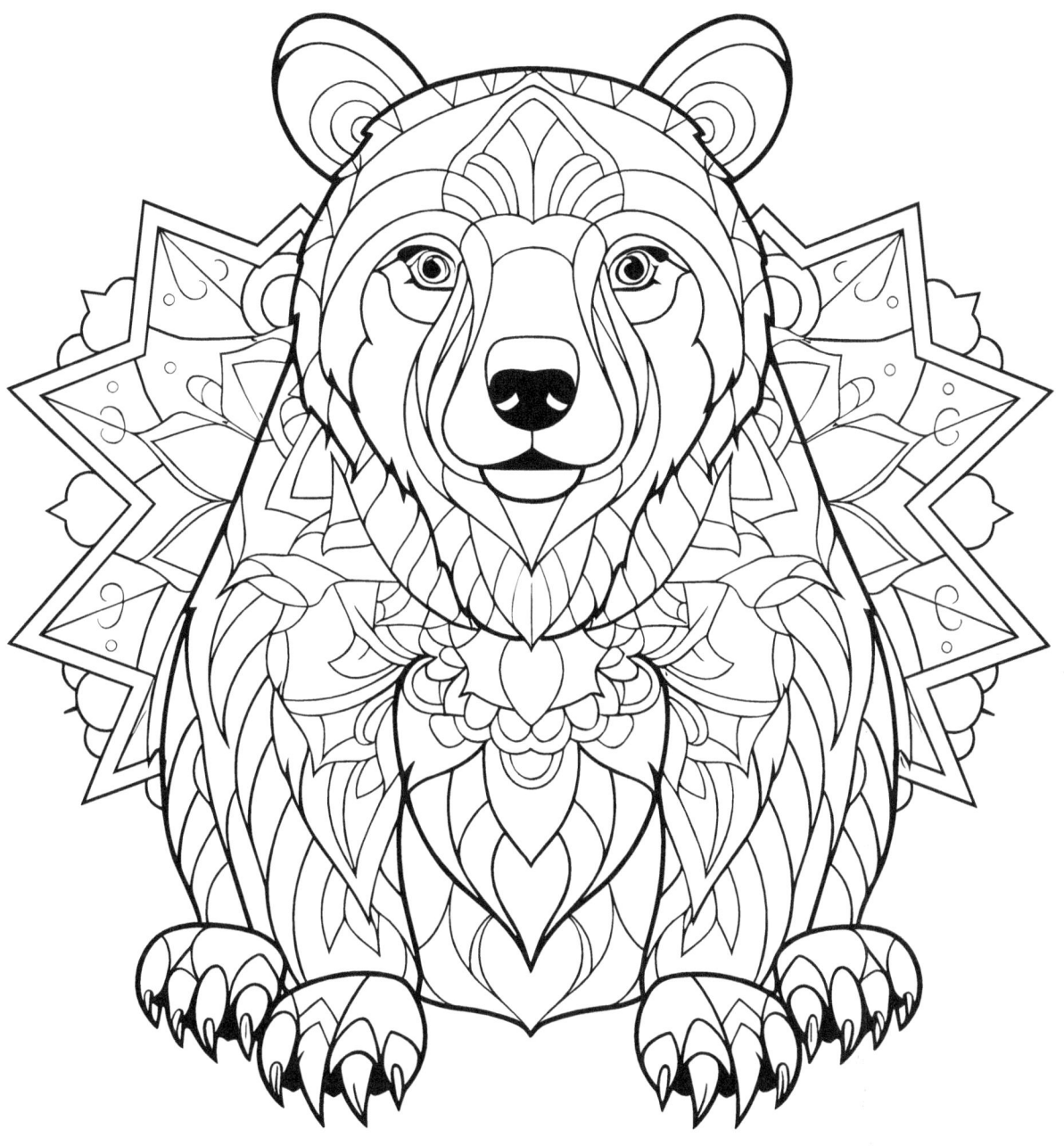

Blank by Design

Balanced Mind Balanced Life

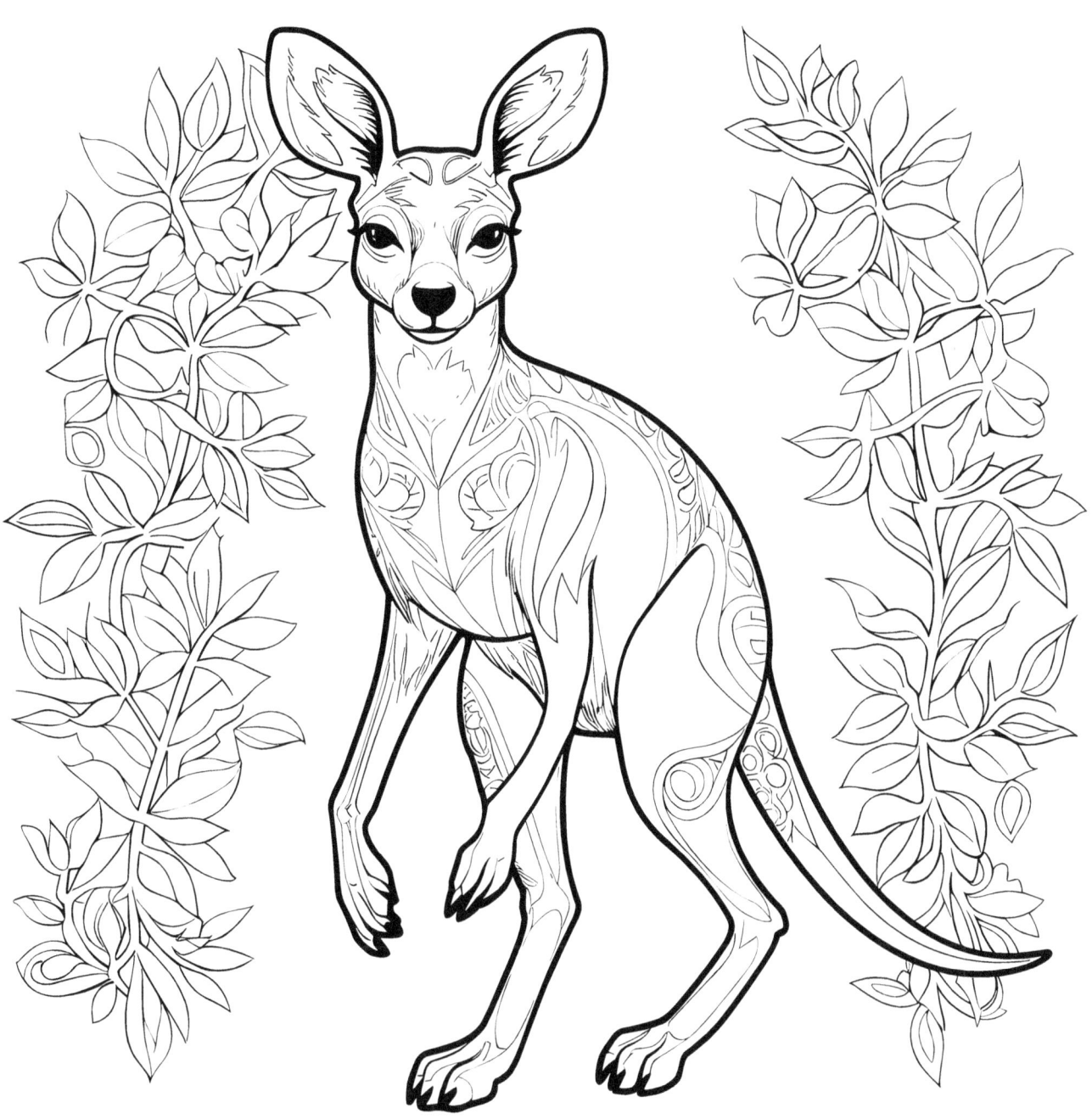

Joe Aguilus

Blank by Design

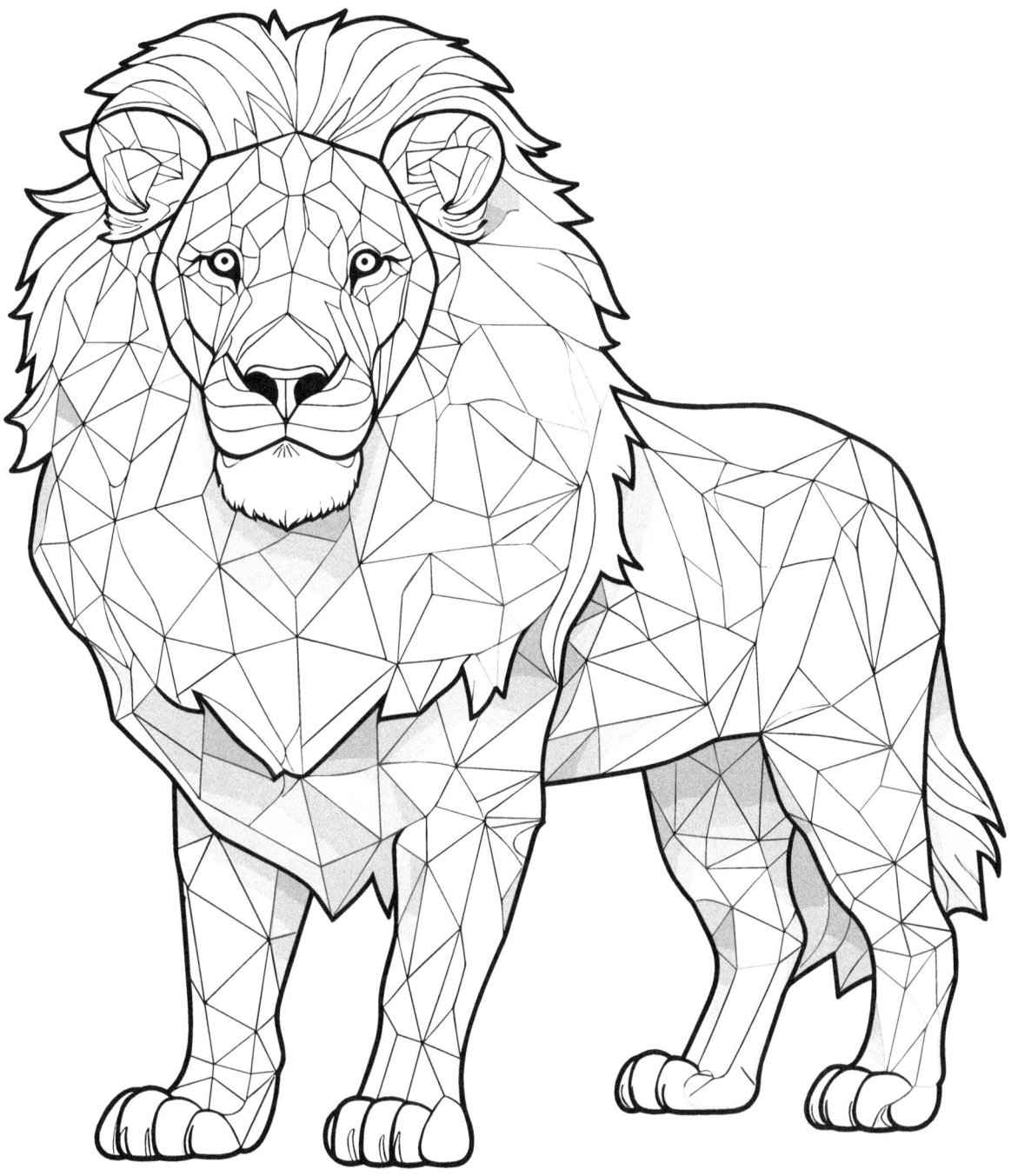

Blank by Design

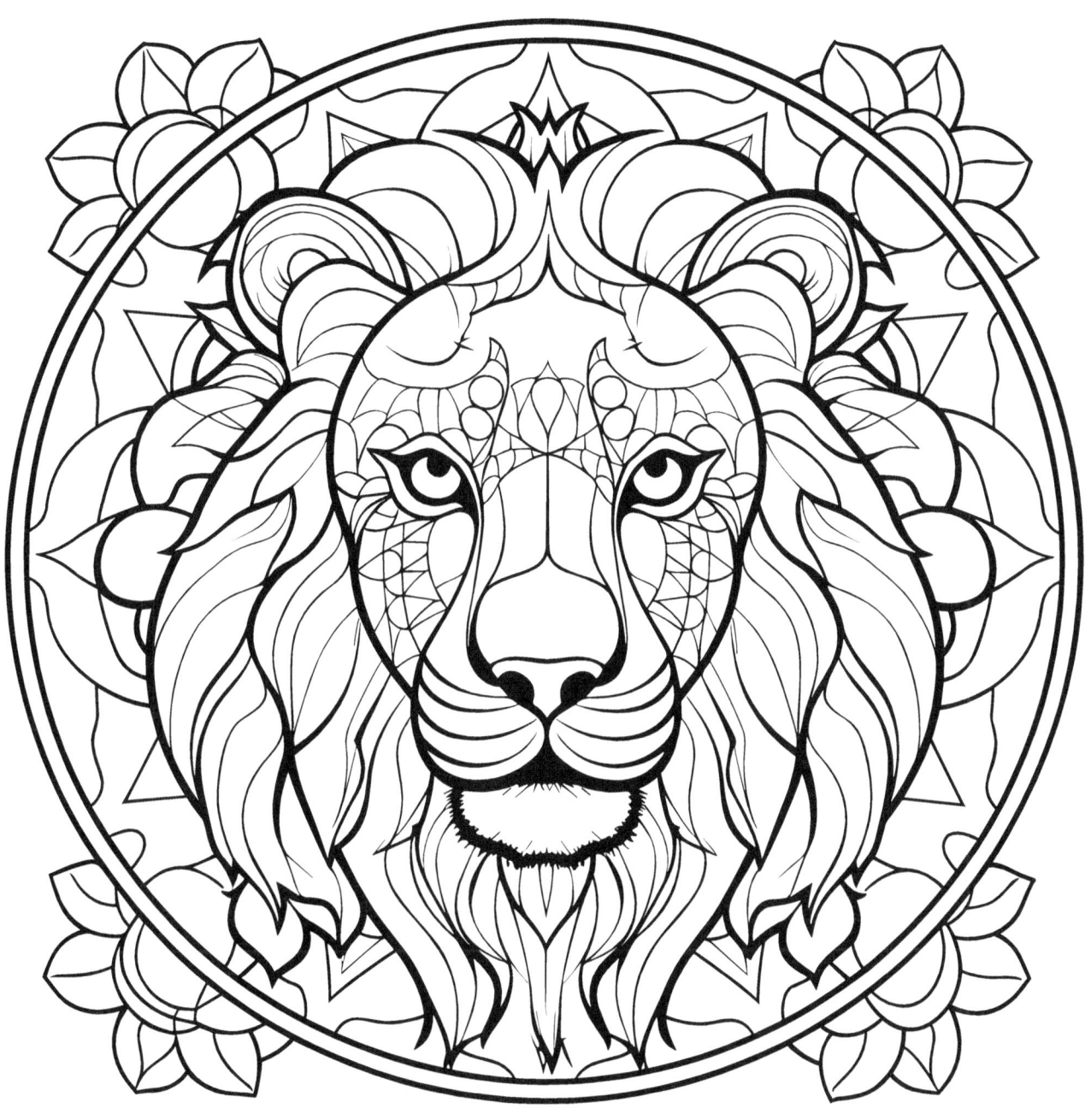

Joe Aguilus

*Blank by
Design*

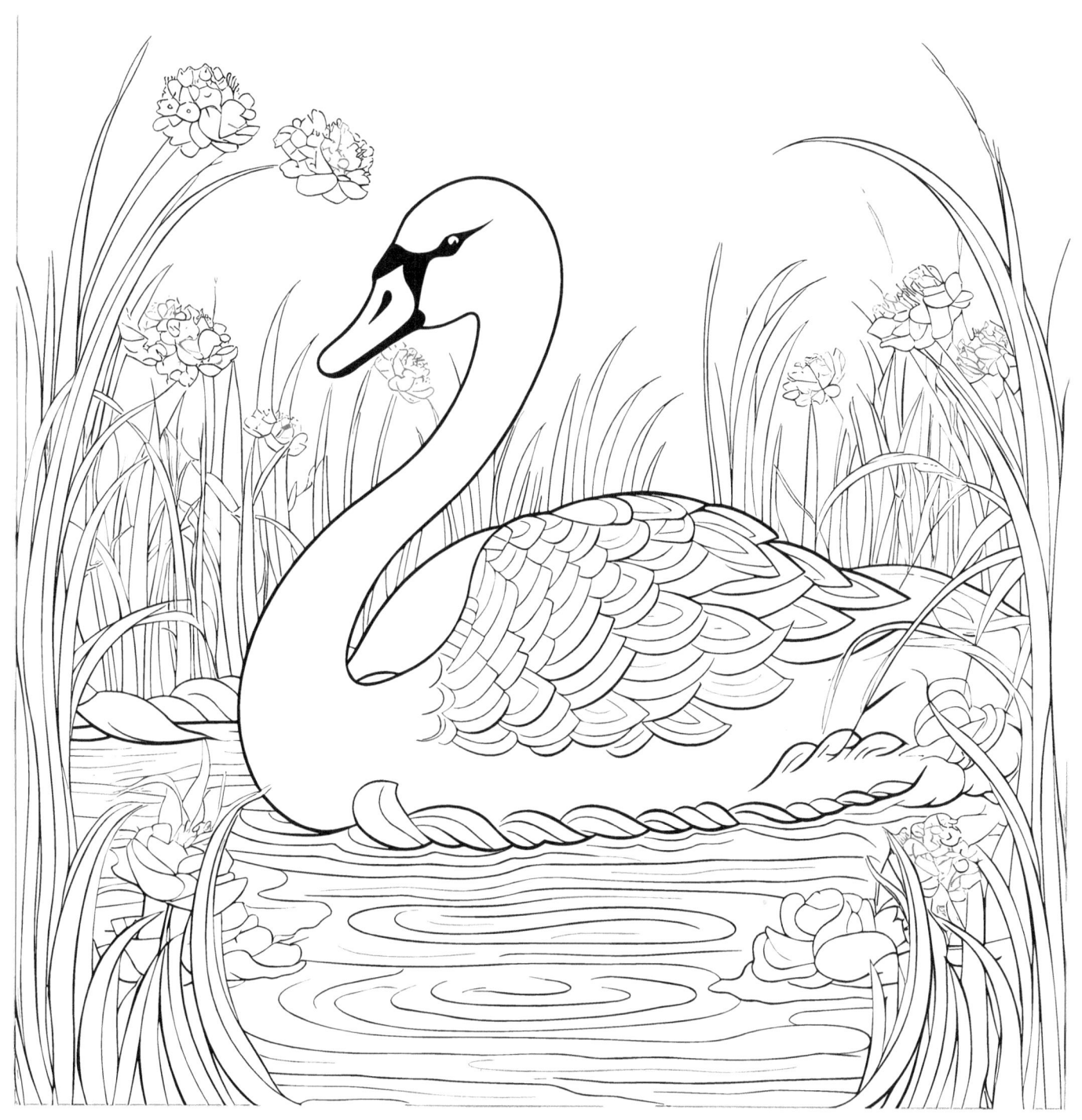

Blank by Design

Balanced Mind Balanced Life

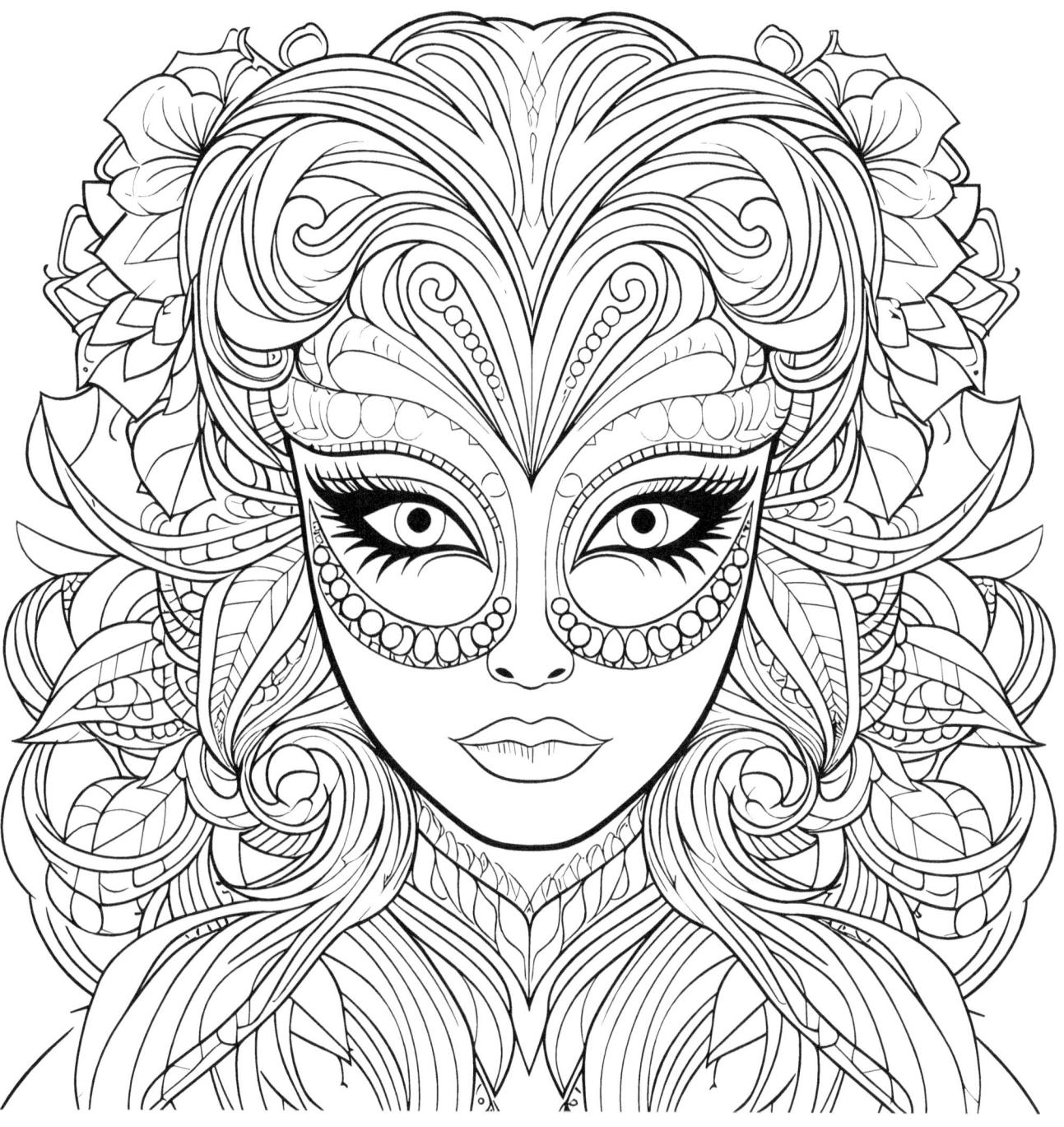

Joe Aguilus

Blank by Design

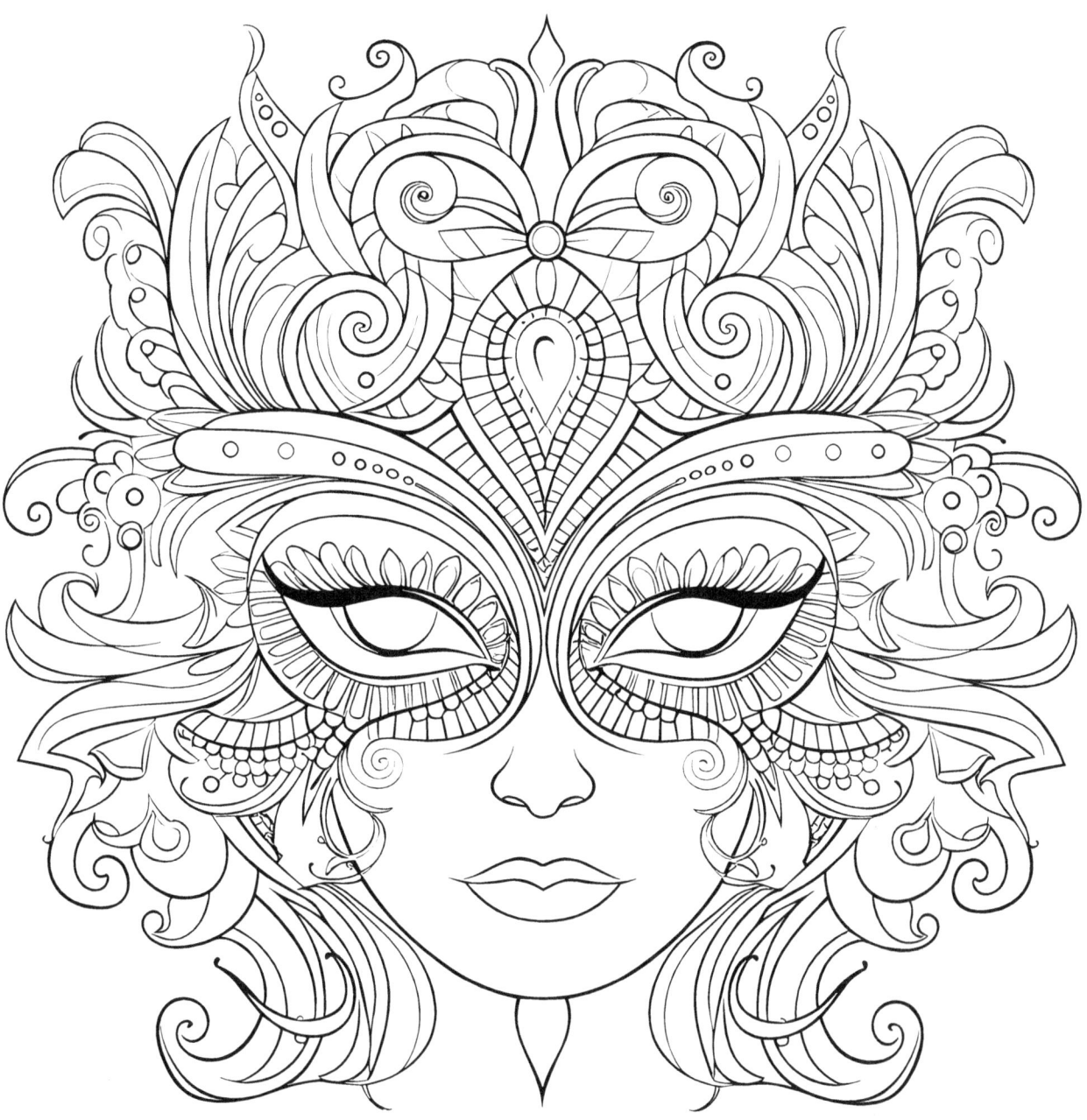

Blank by Design

Balanced Mind Balanced Life

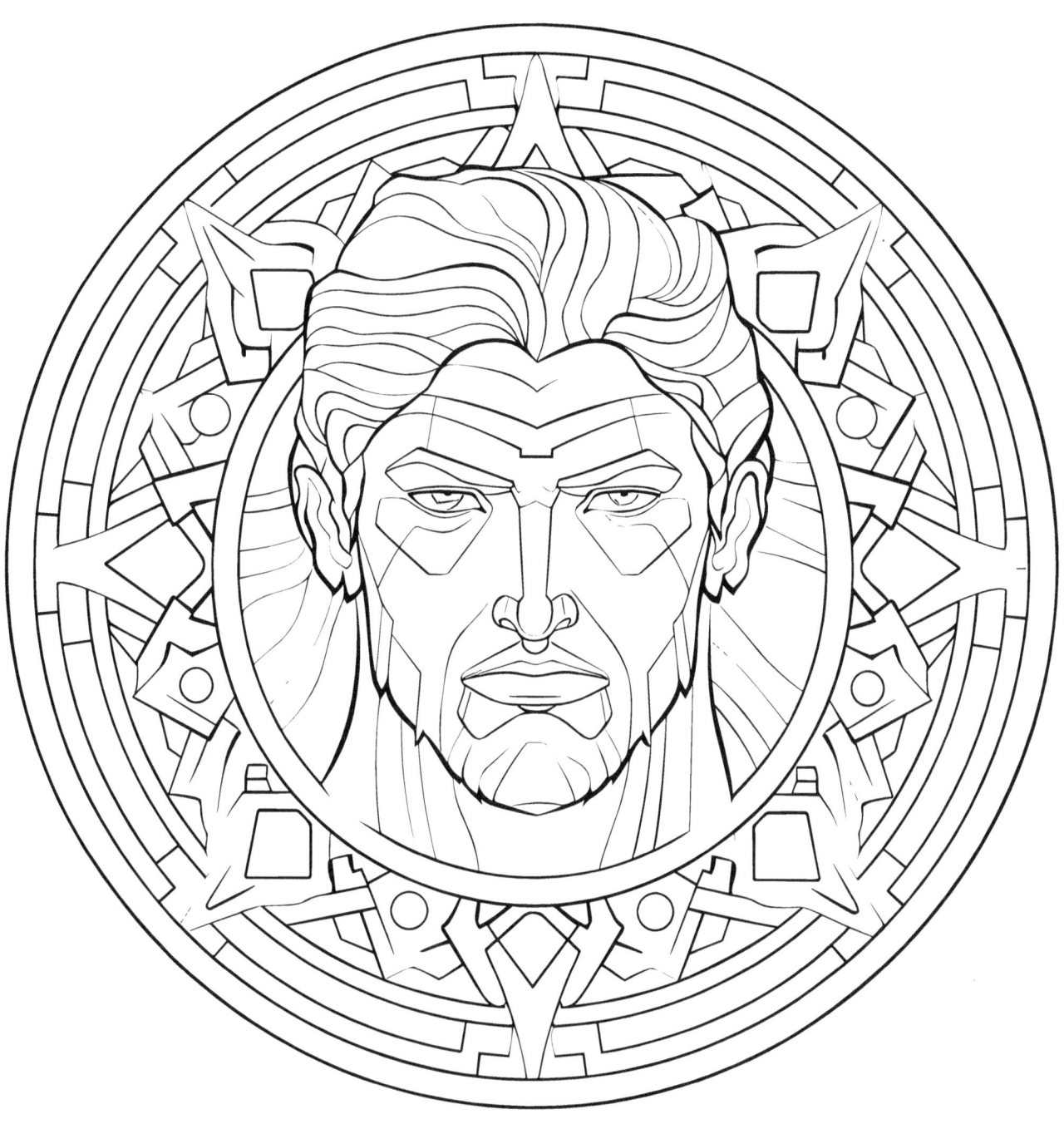

Blank by Design

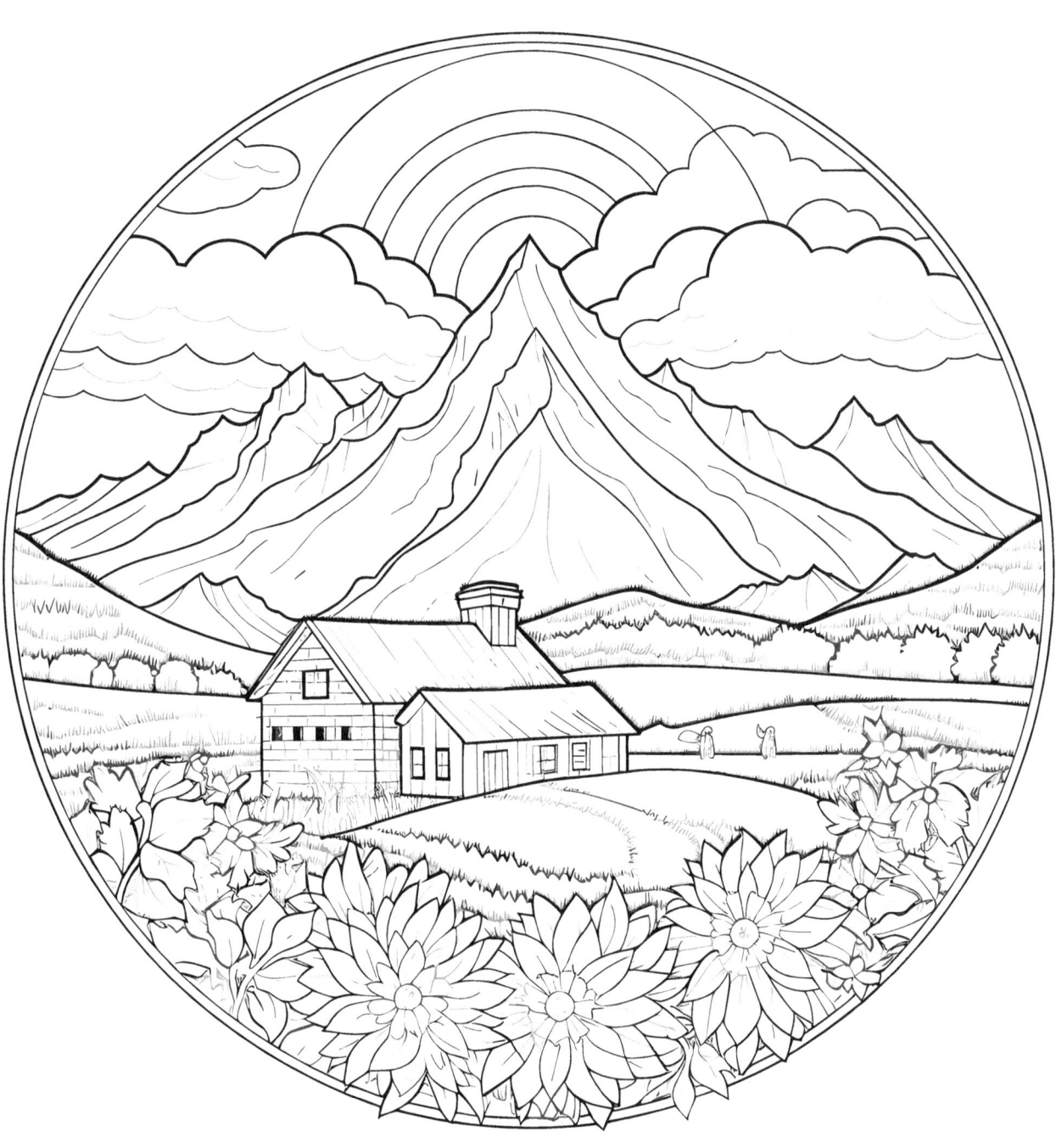

Blank by Design

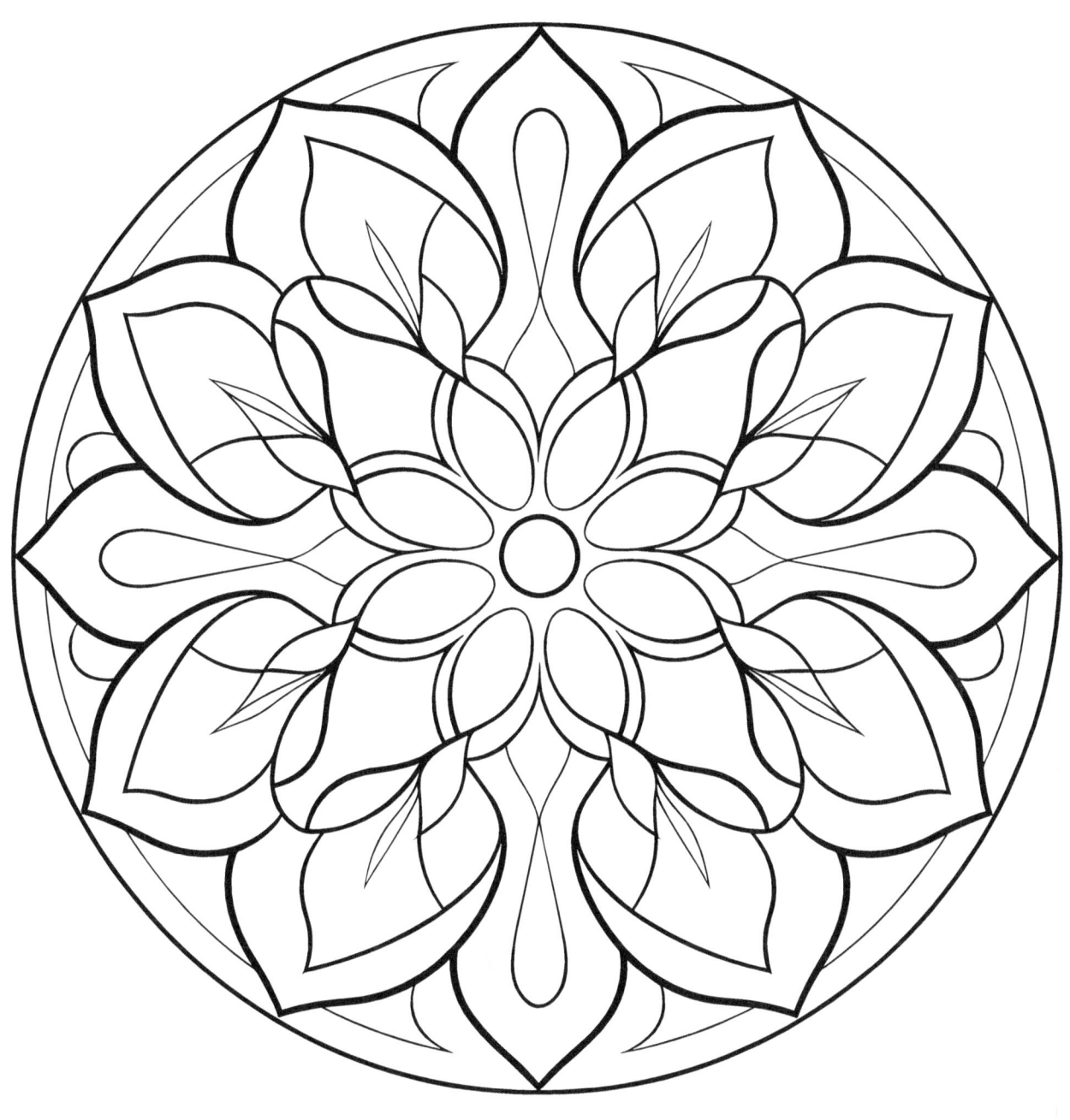

Joe Aguilus

Blank by Design

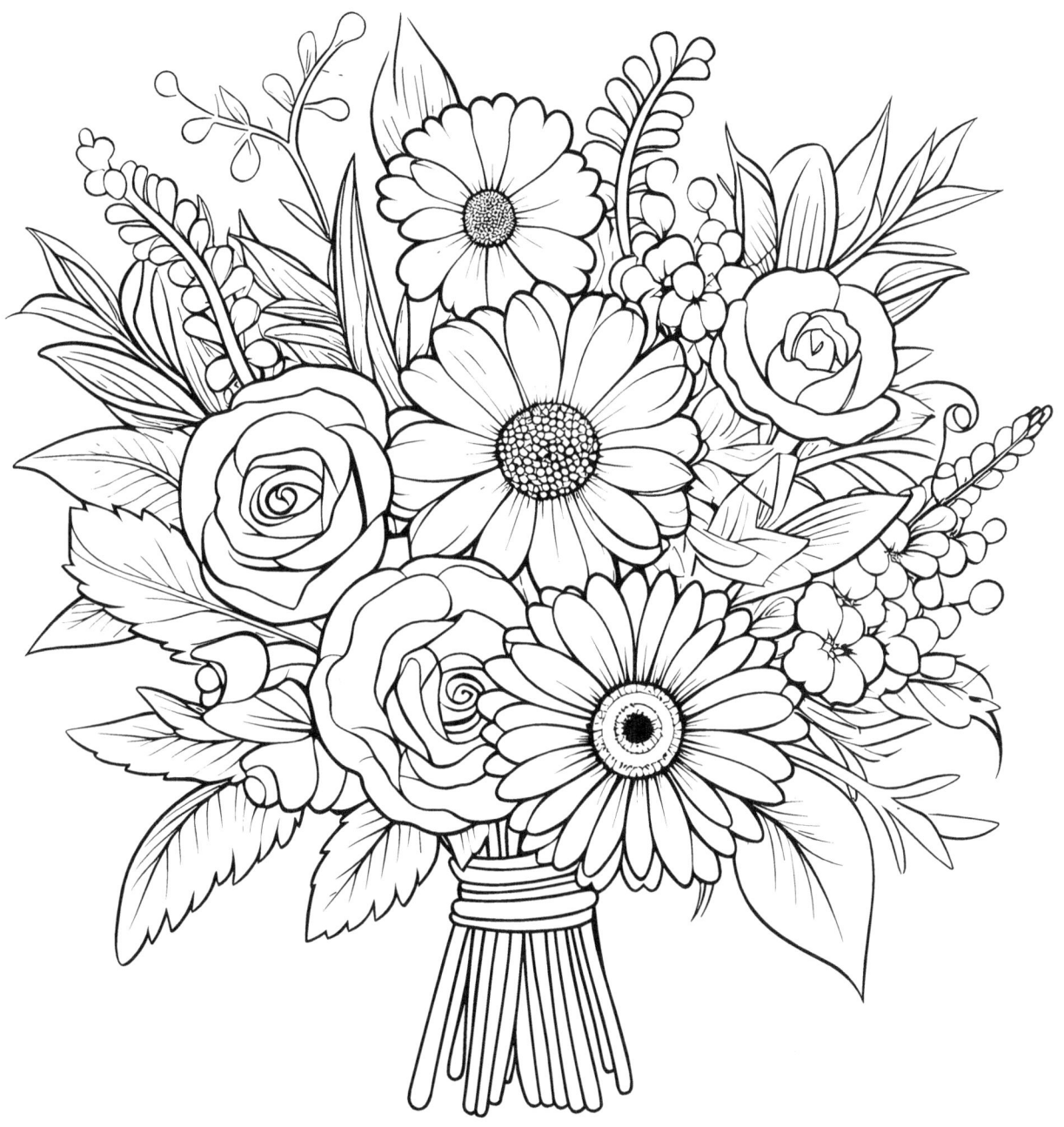

Blank by Design

Balanced Mind Balanced Life

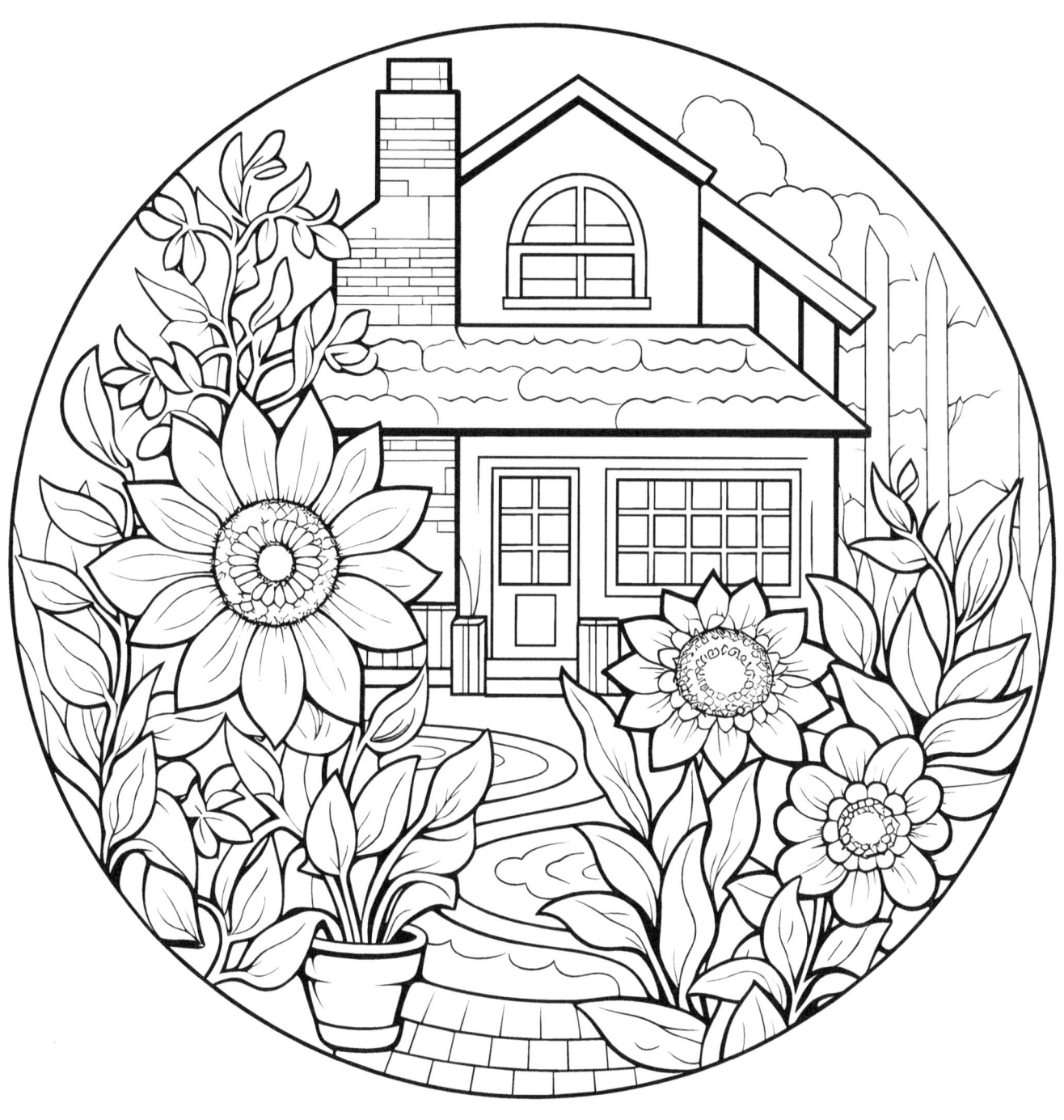

Blank by Design

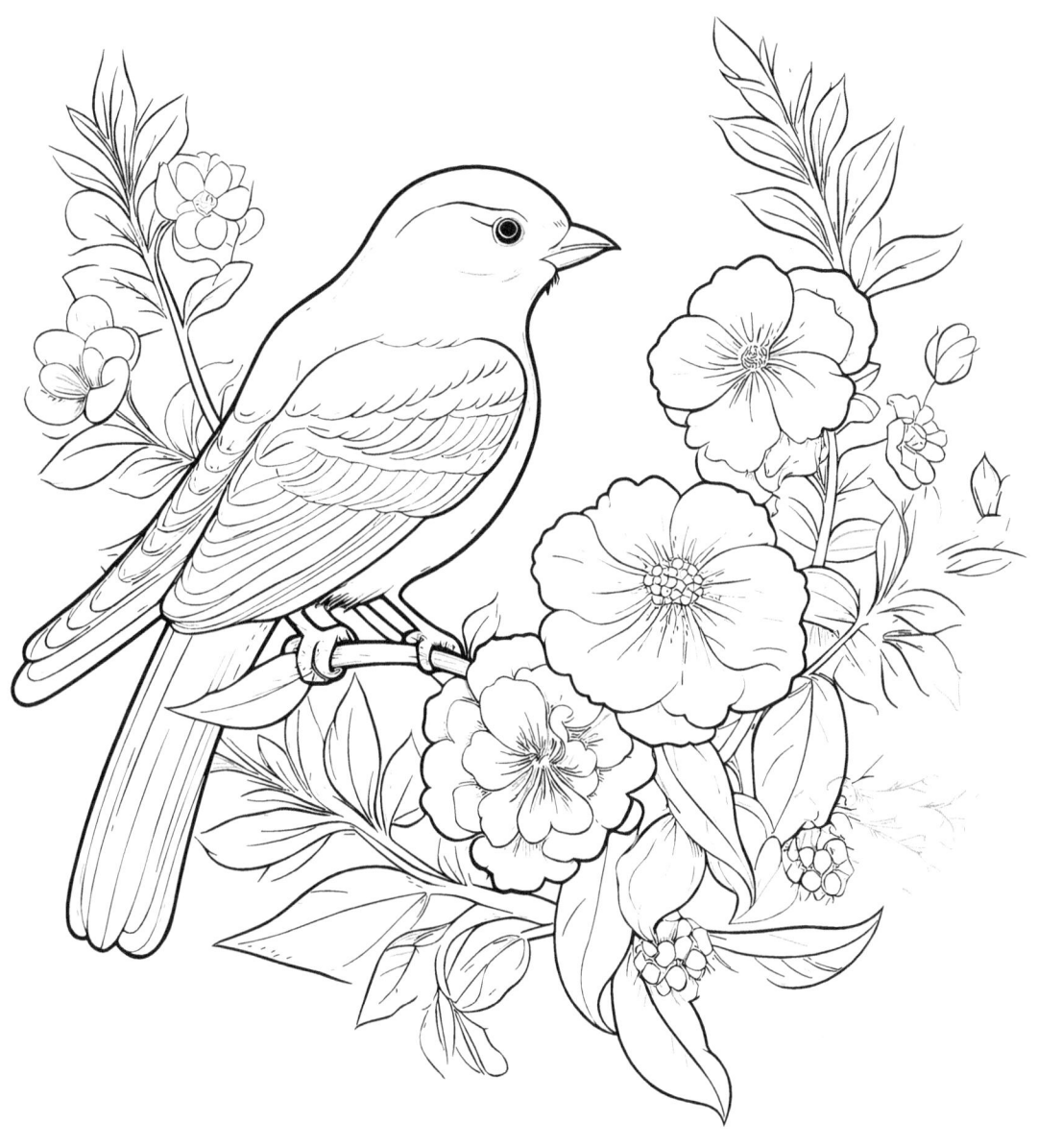

Blank by Design

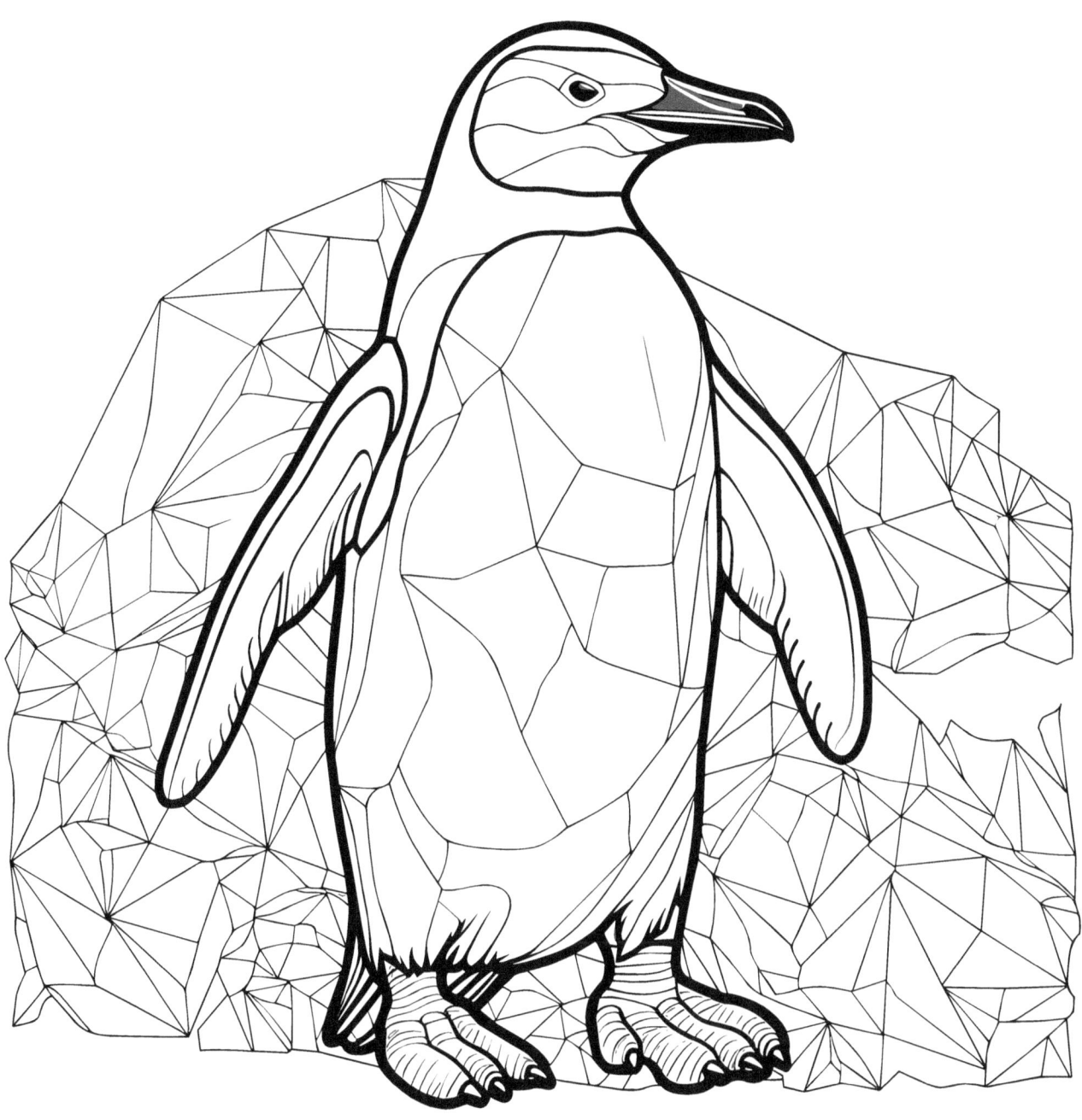

Joe Aguilus

*Blank by
Design*

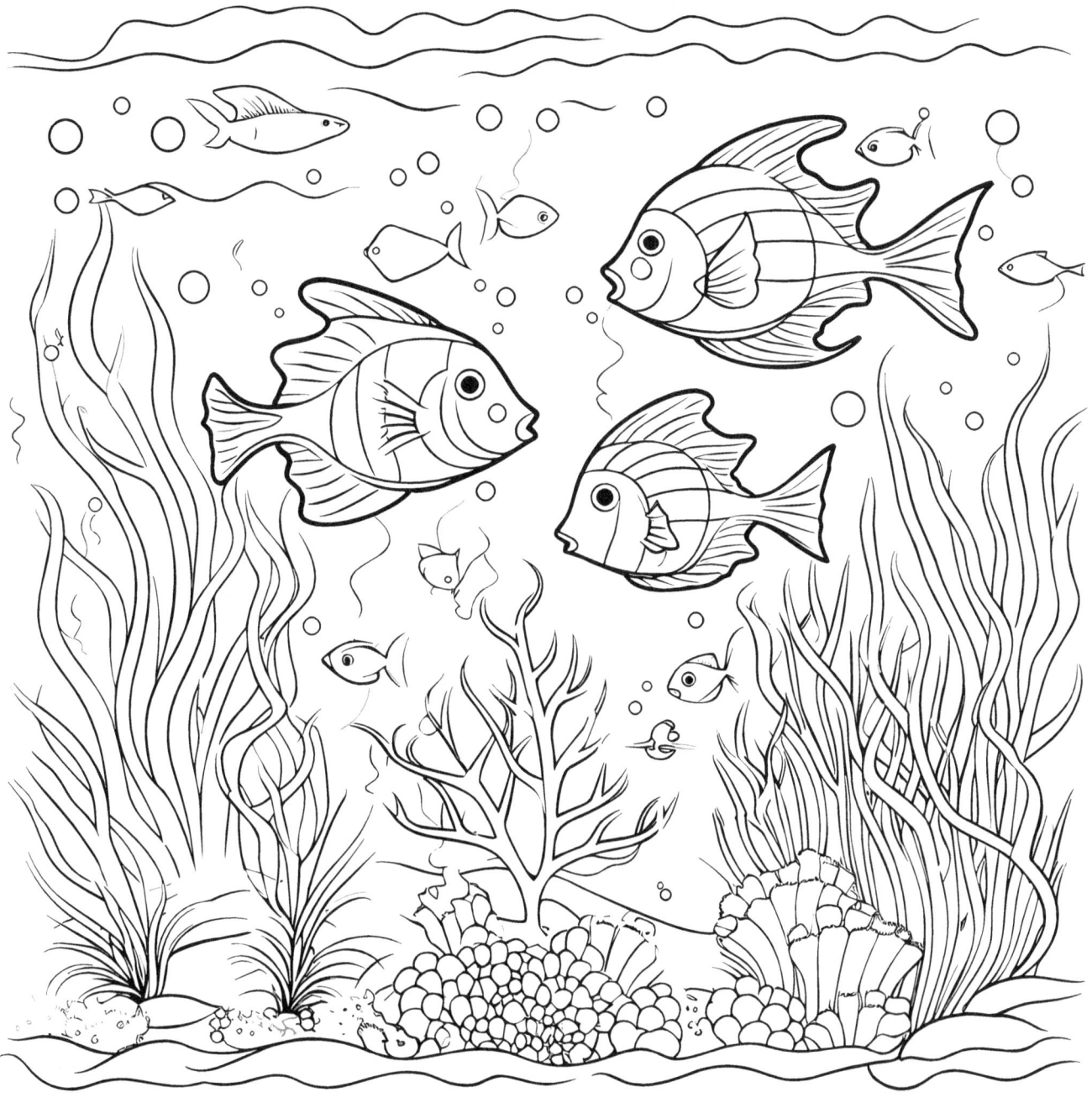

Blank by Design

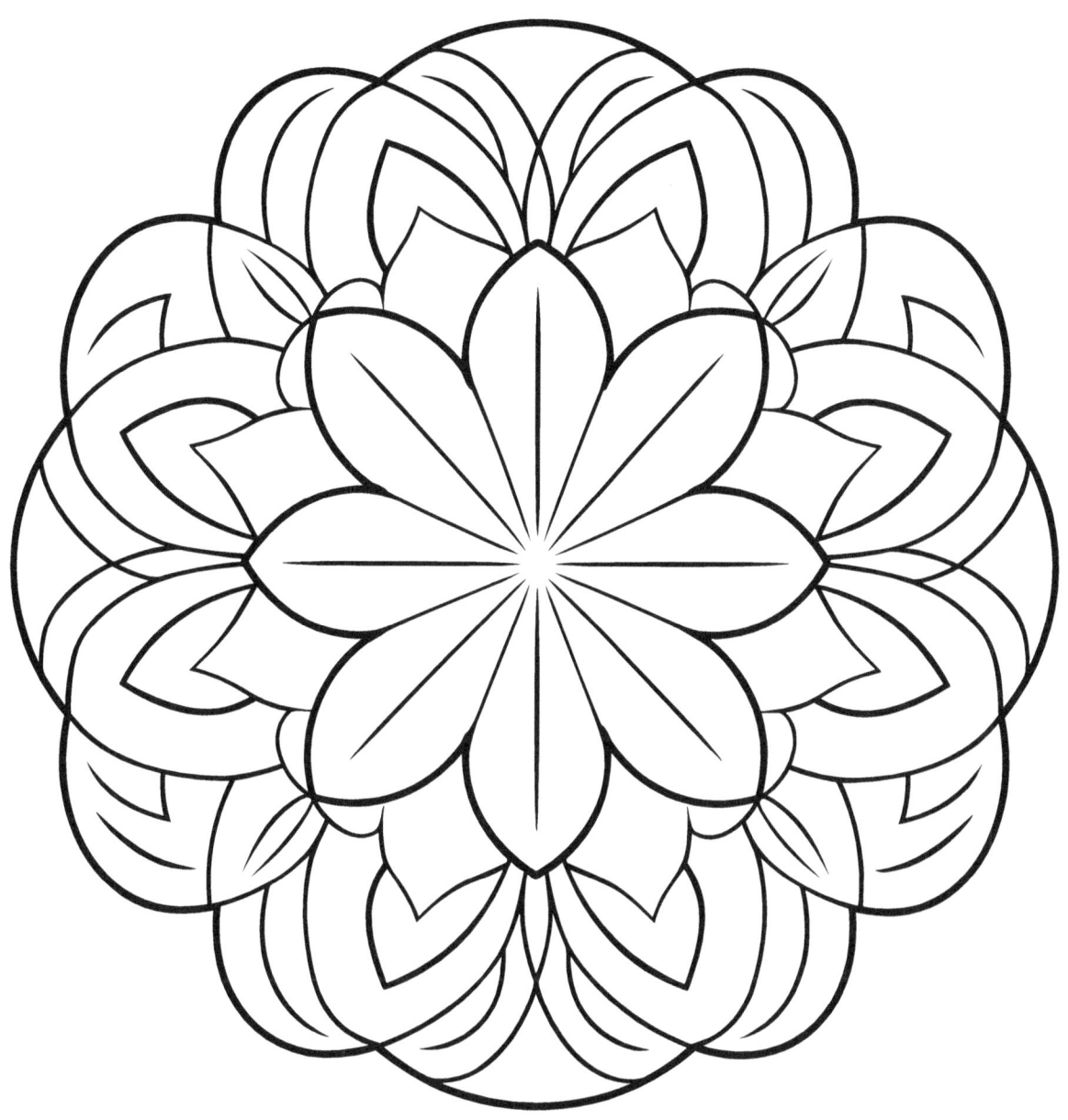

Joe Aguilus

*Blank by
Design*

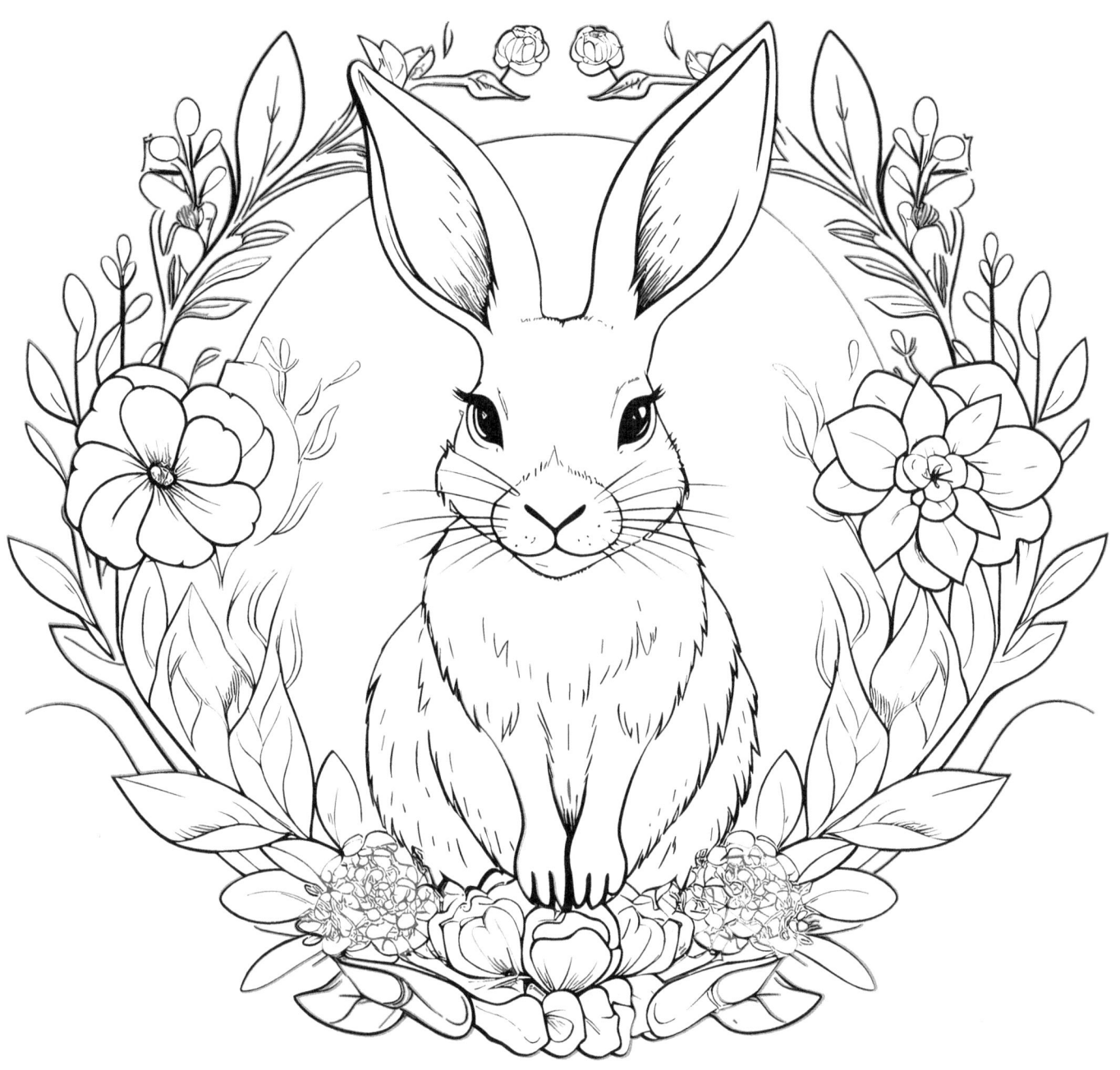

Blank by Design

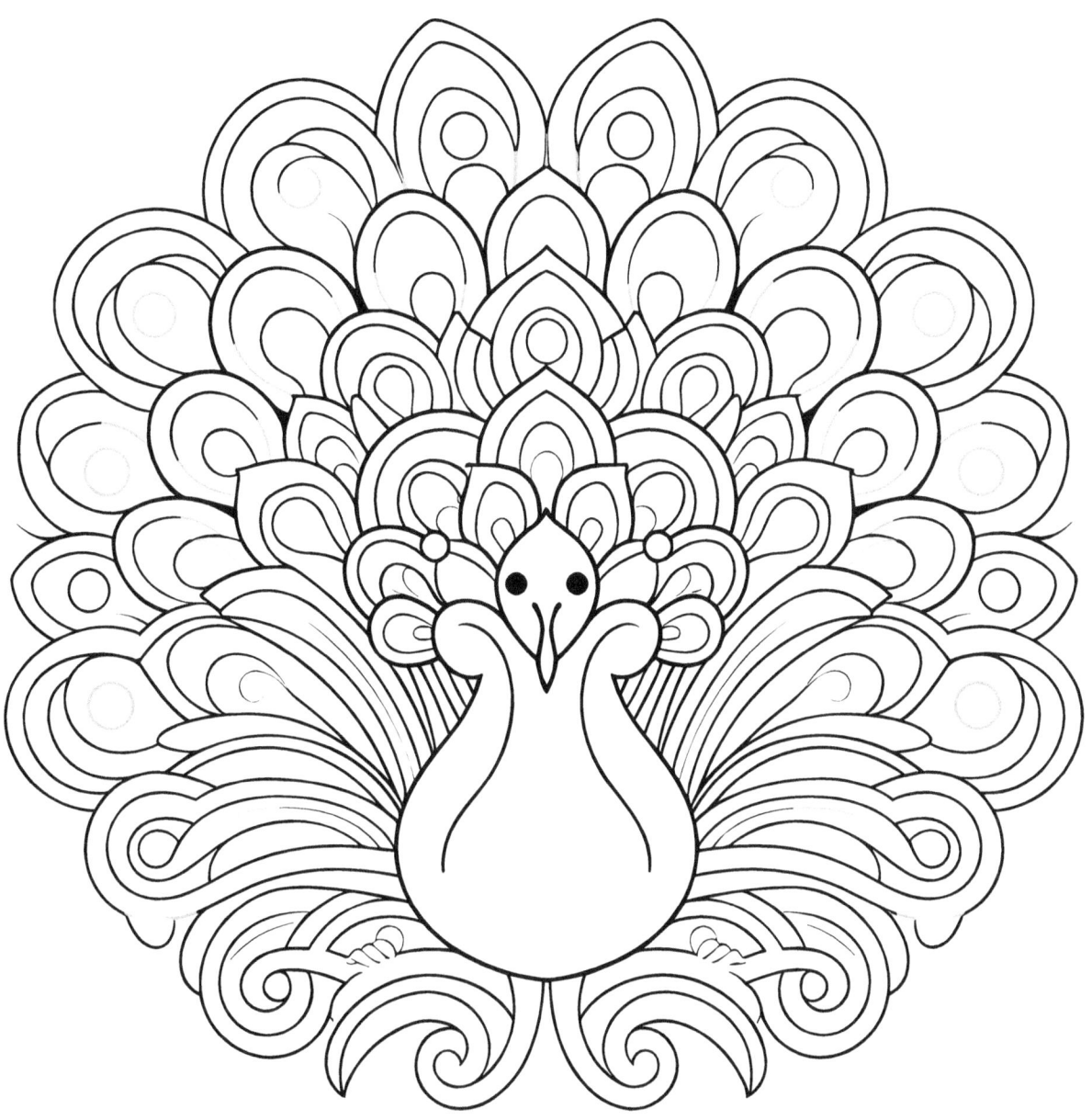

Blank by Design

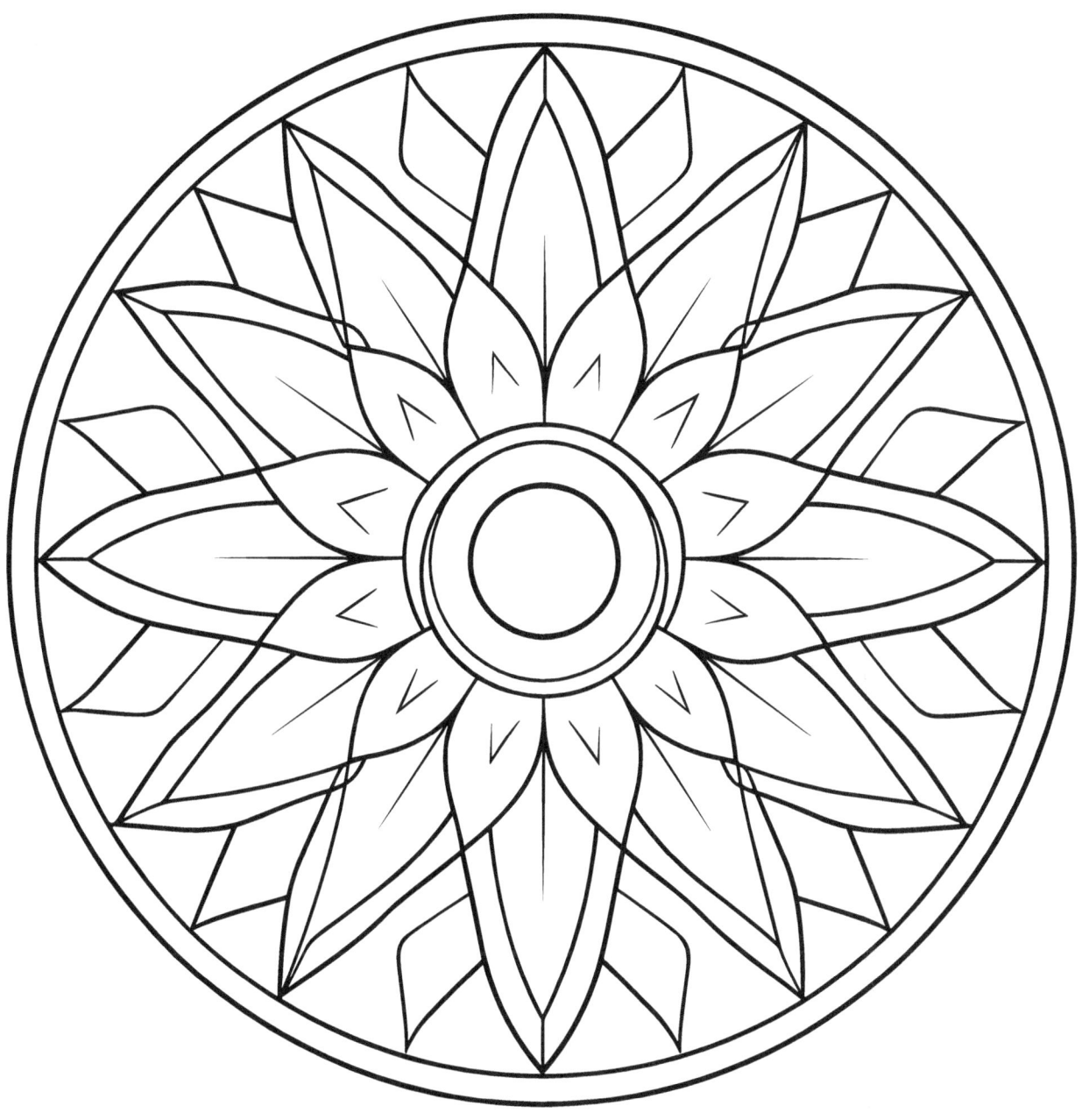

Blank by Design

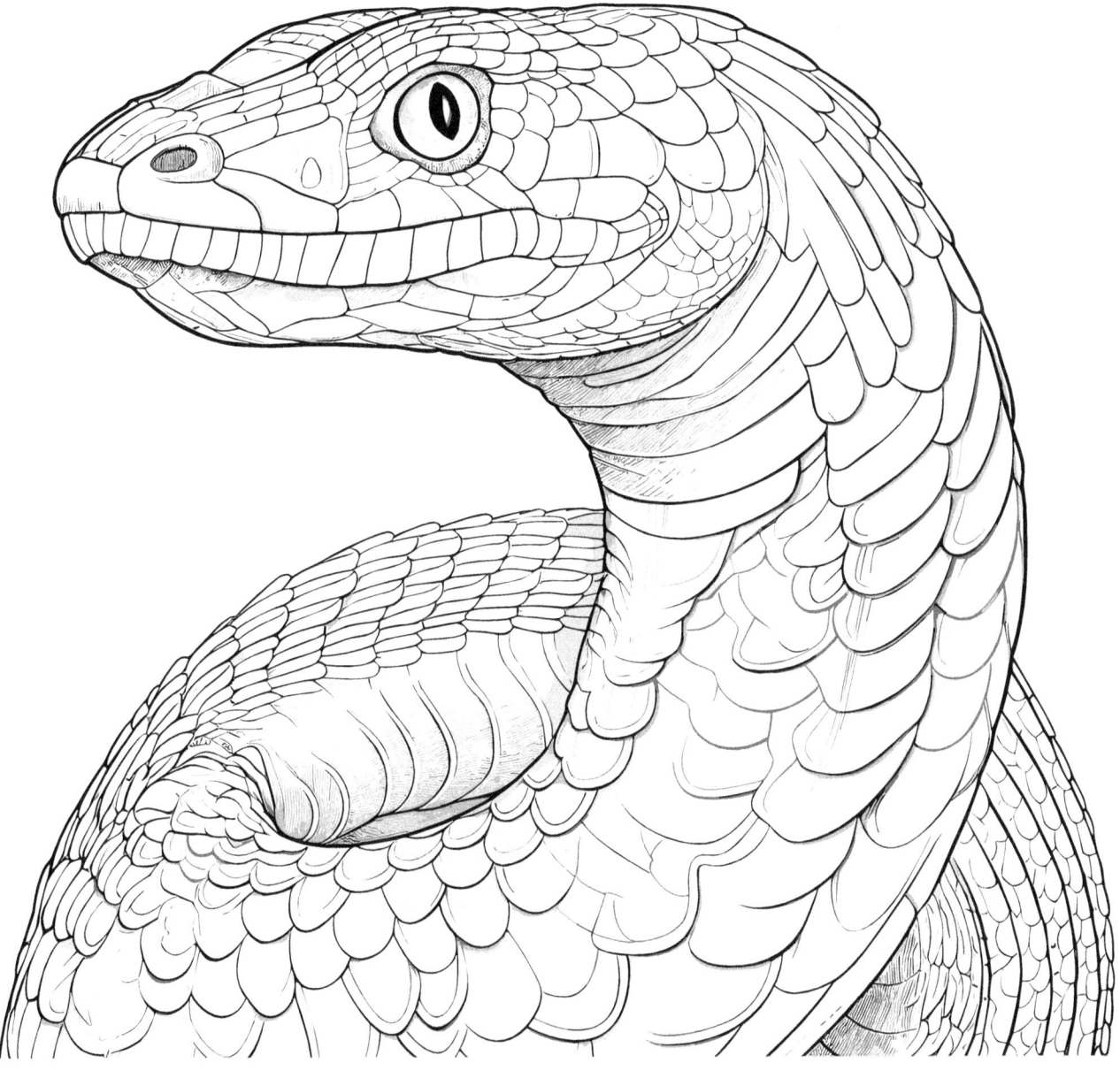

Blank by Design

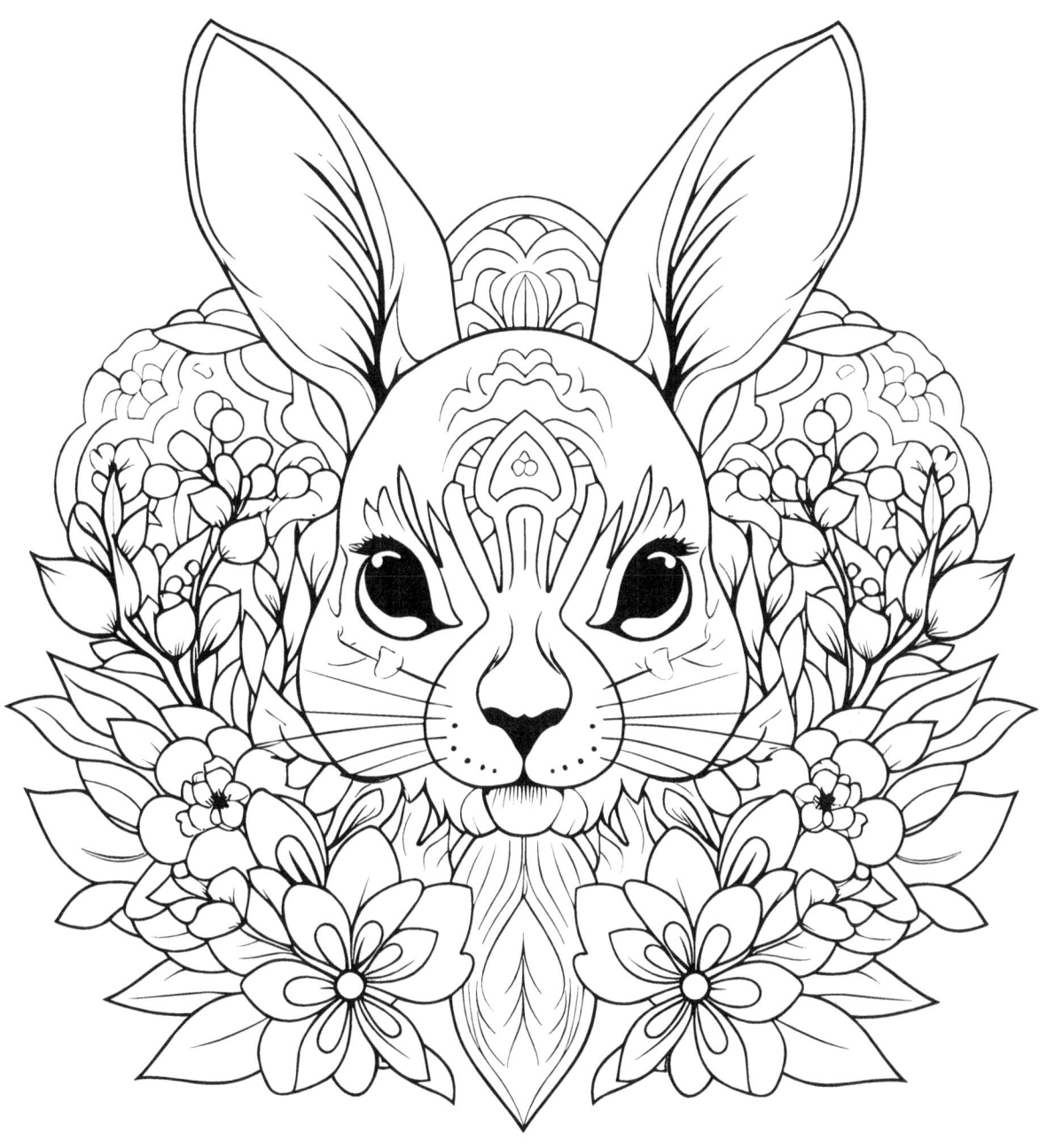

Blank by Design

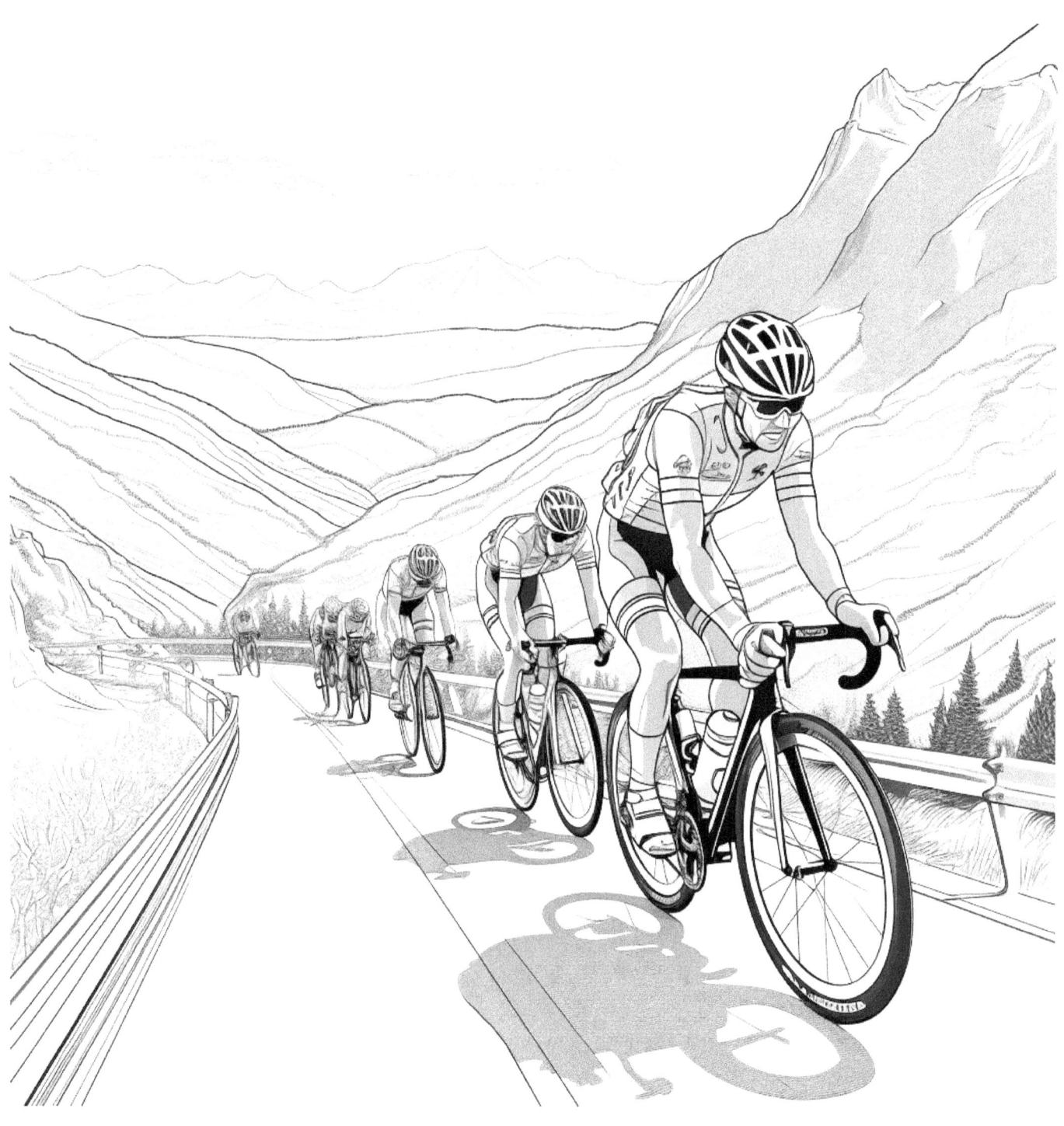

Blank by Design

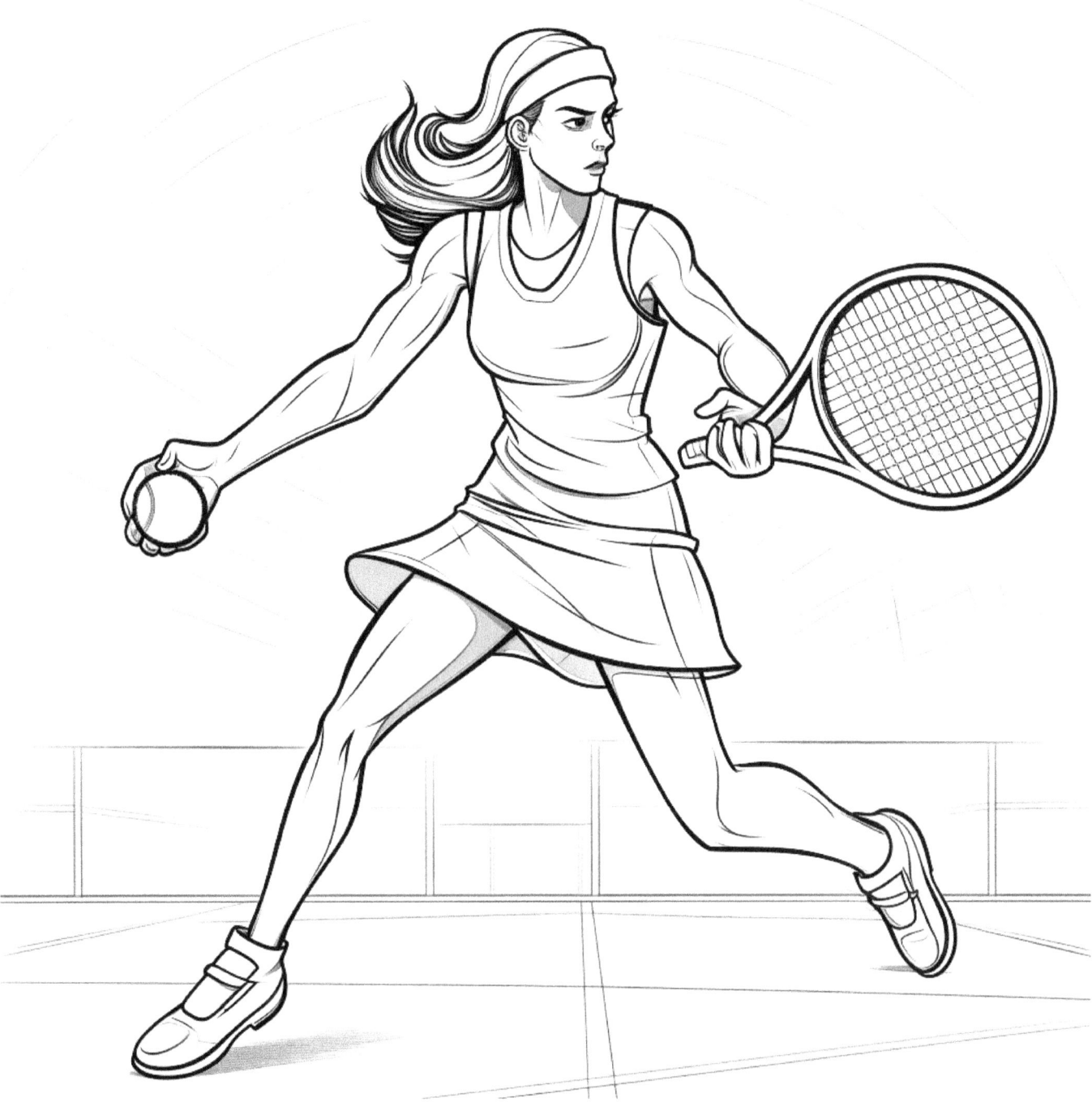

Blank by Design

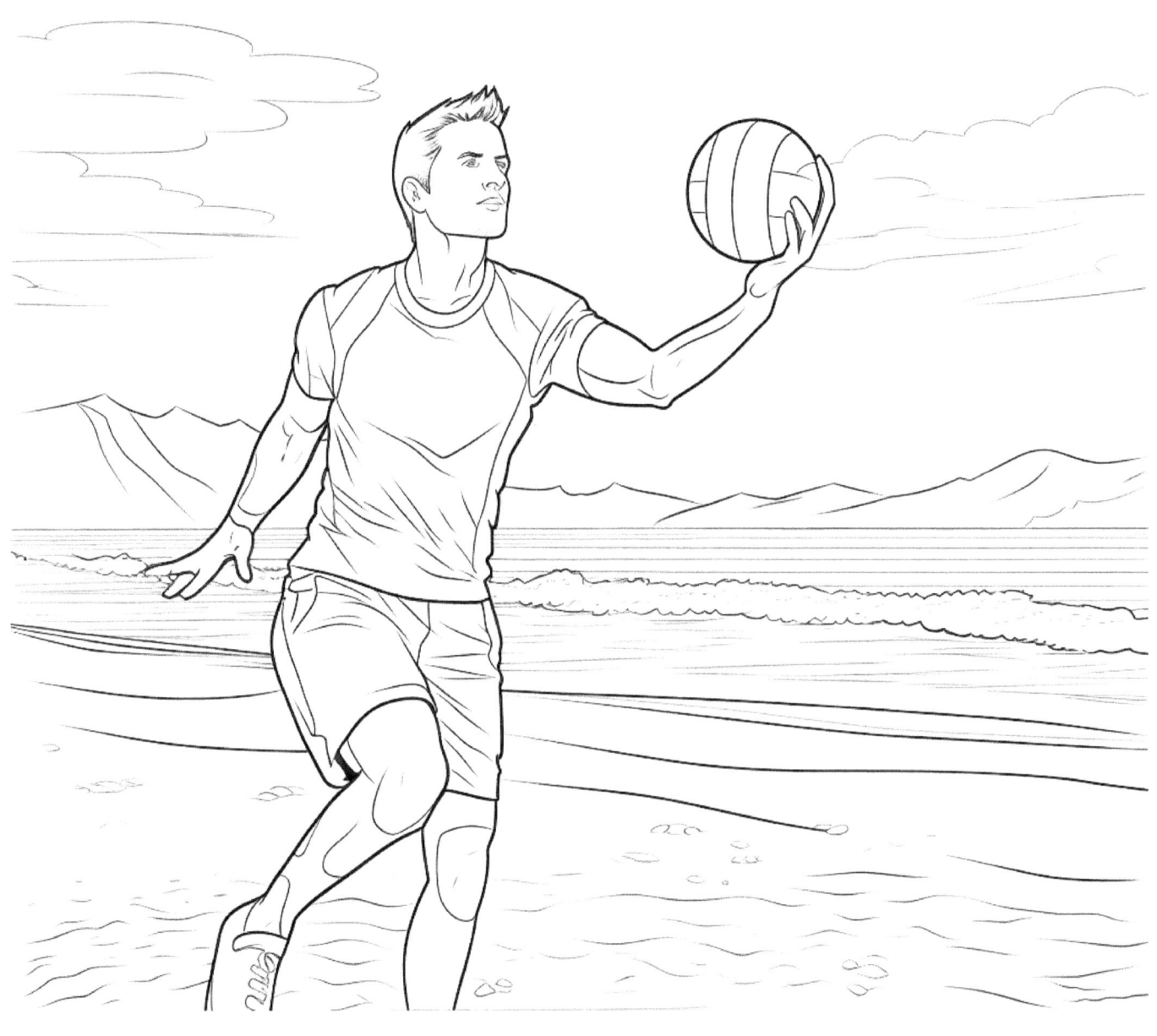

Blank by Design

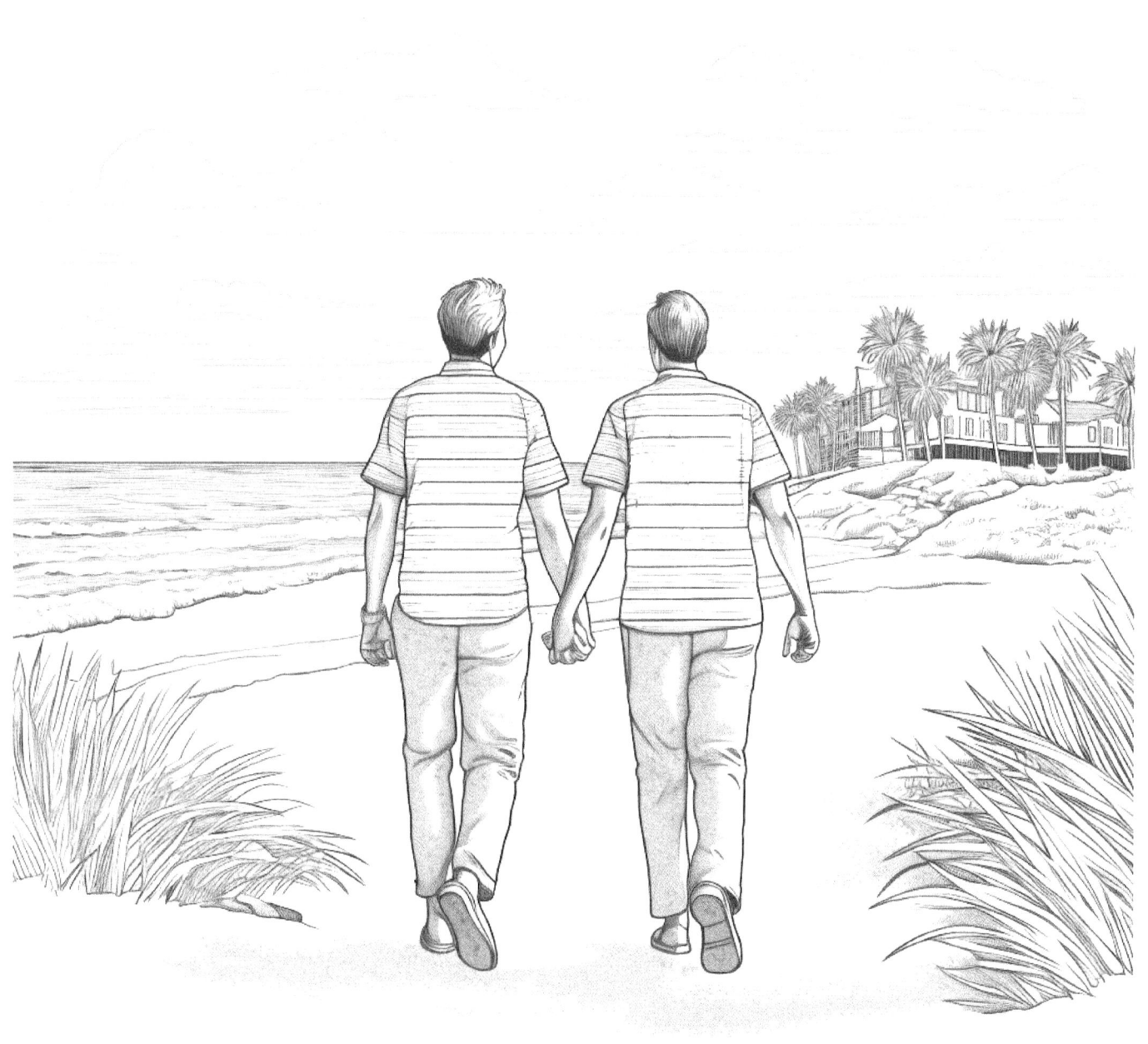

Blank by Design

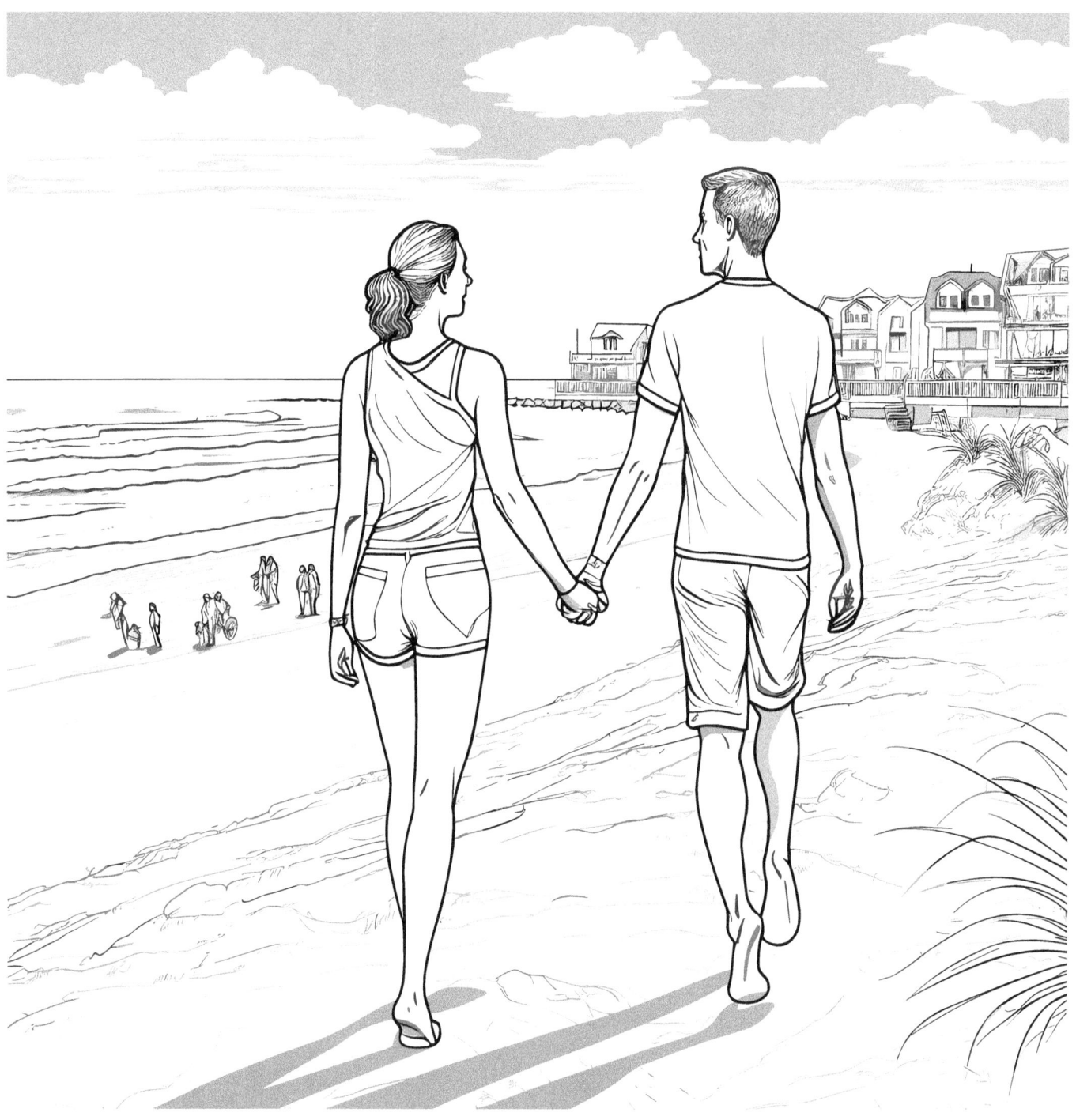

Blank by Design

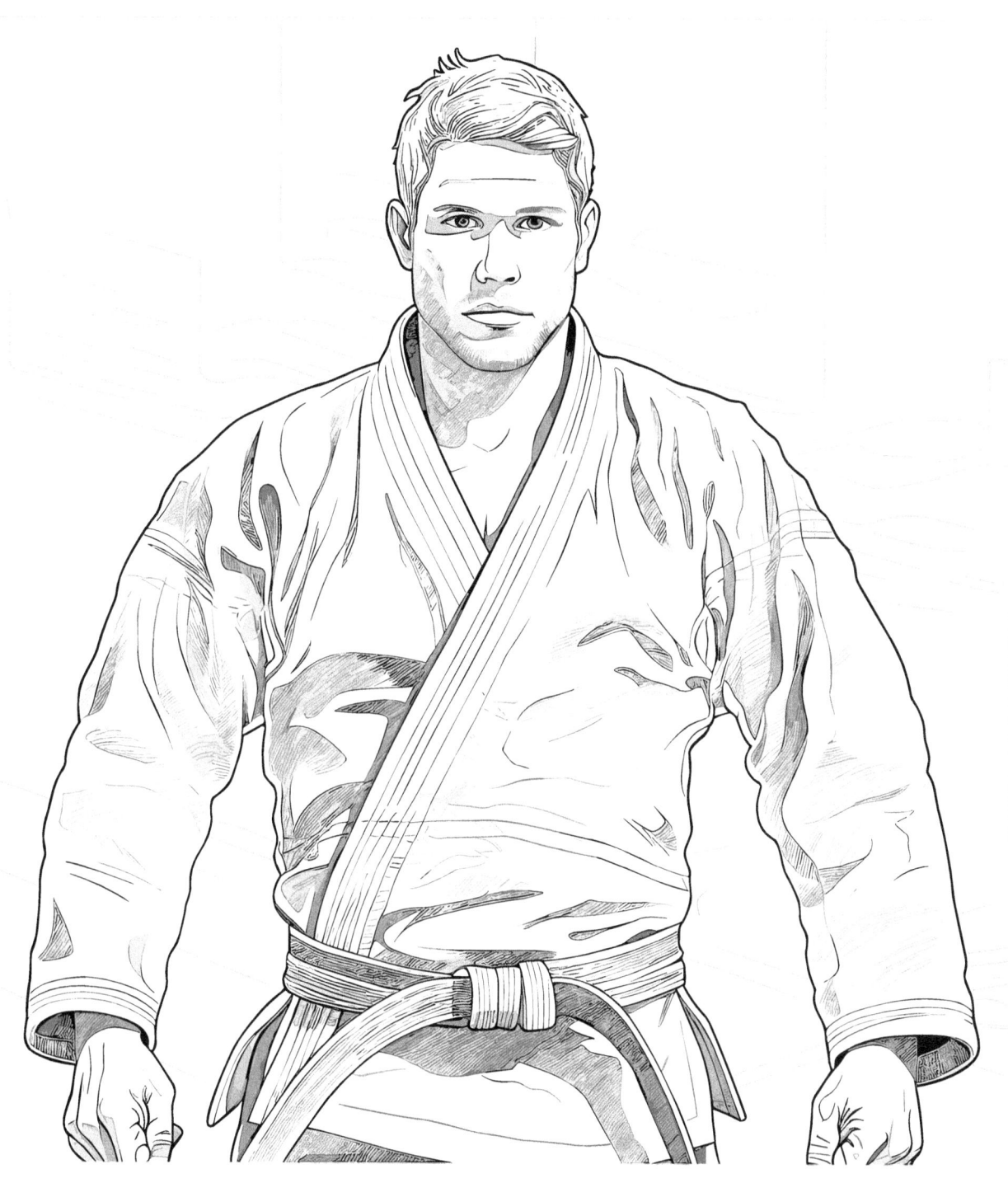

Blank by Design

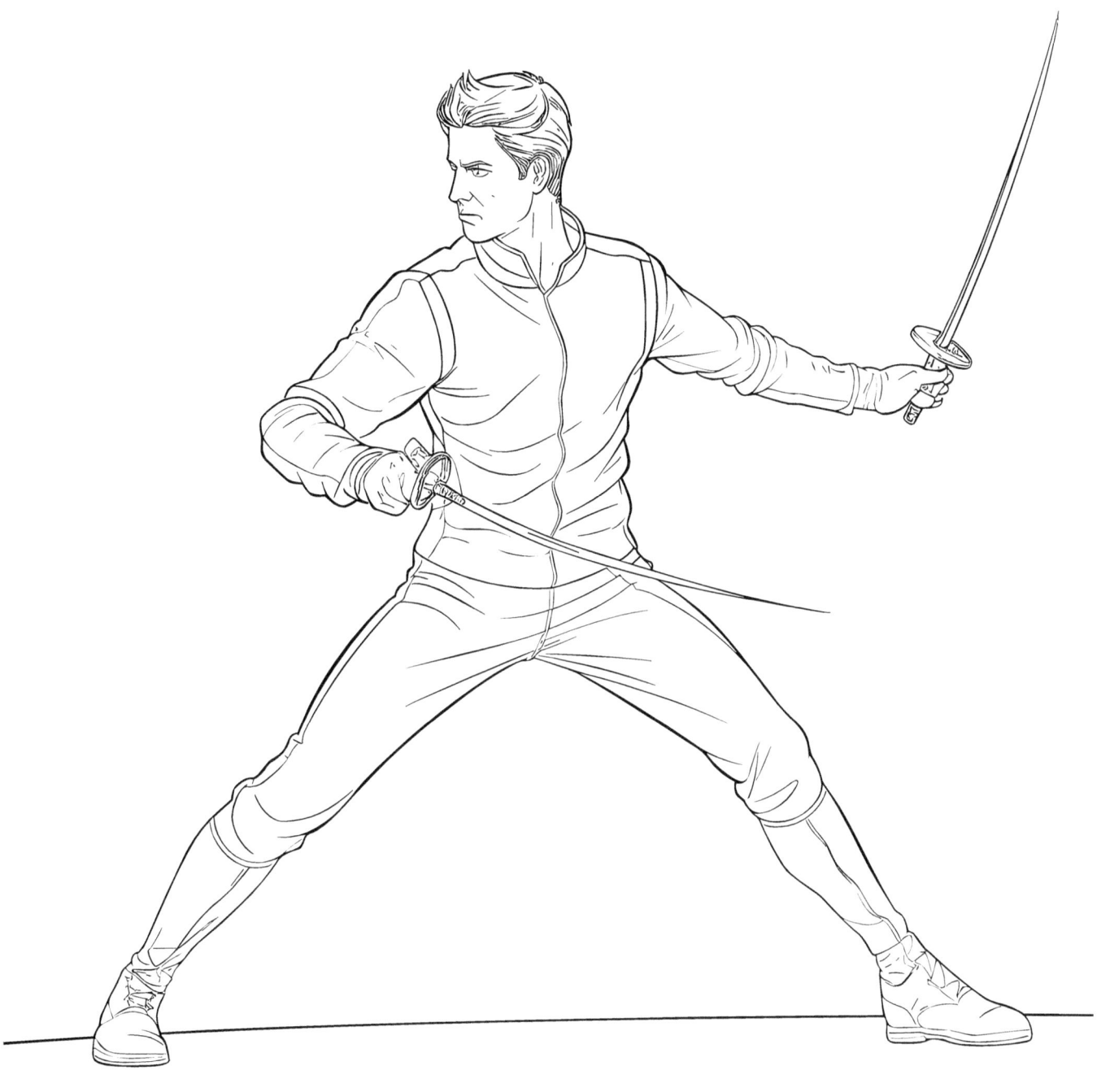

Blank by Design

Balanced Mind Balanced Life

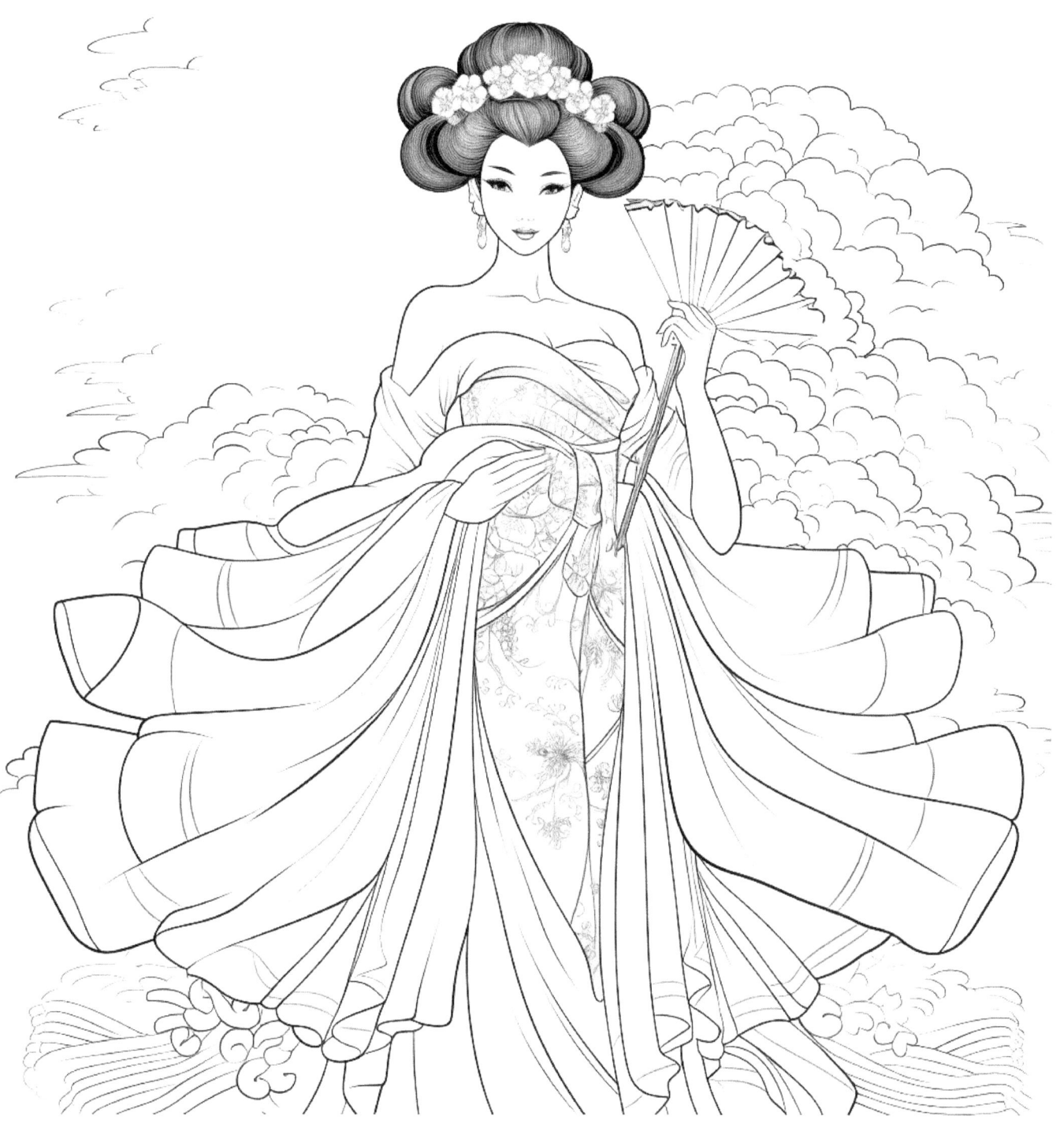

Blank by Design

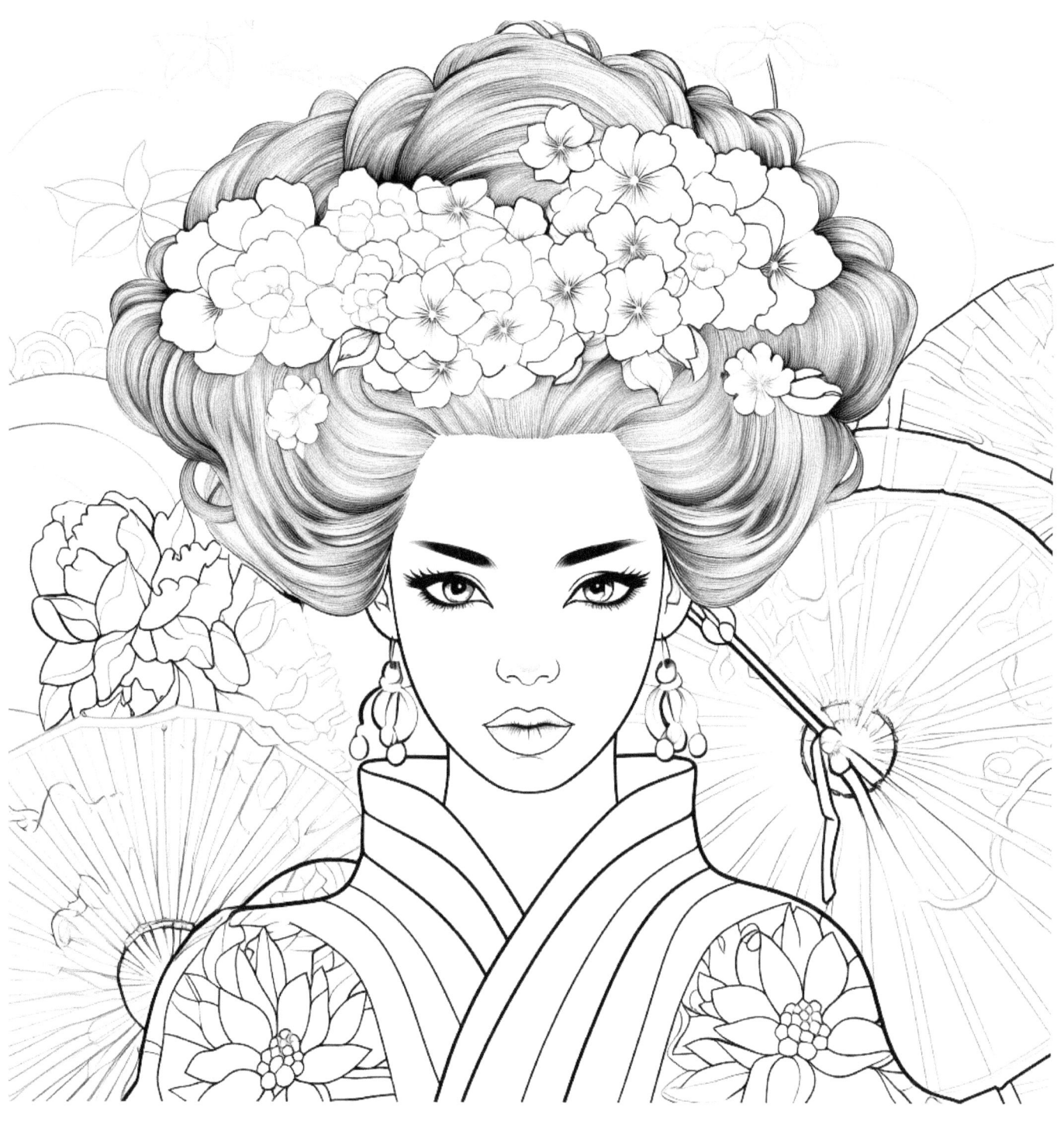

Blank by Design

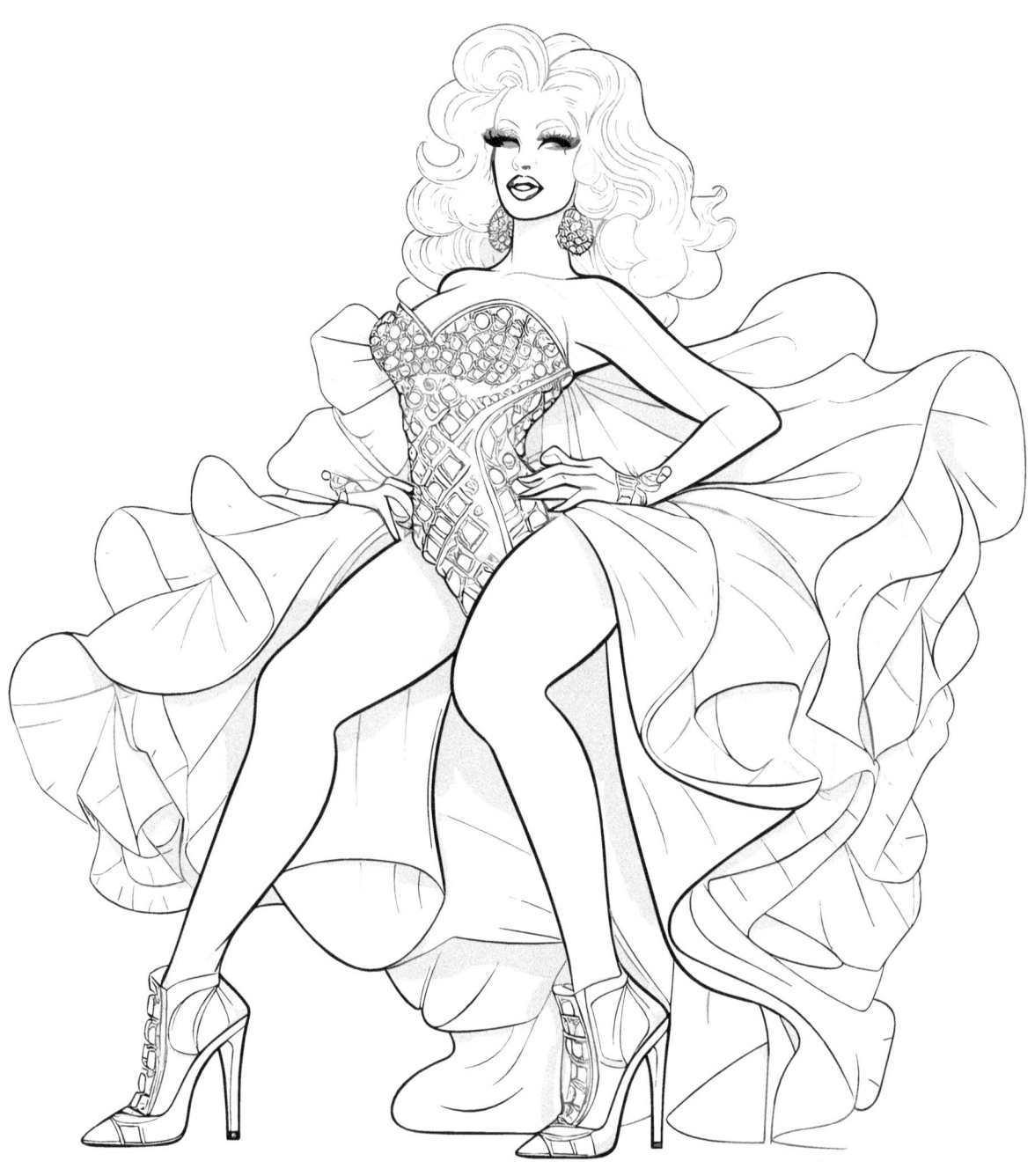

Blank by Design

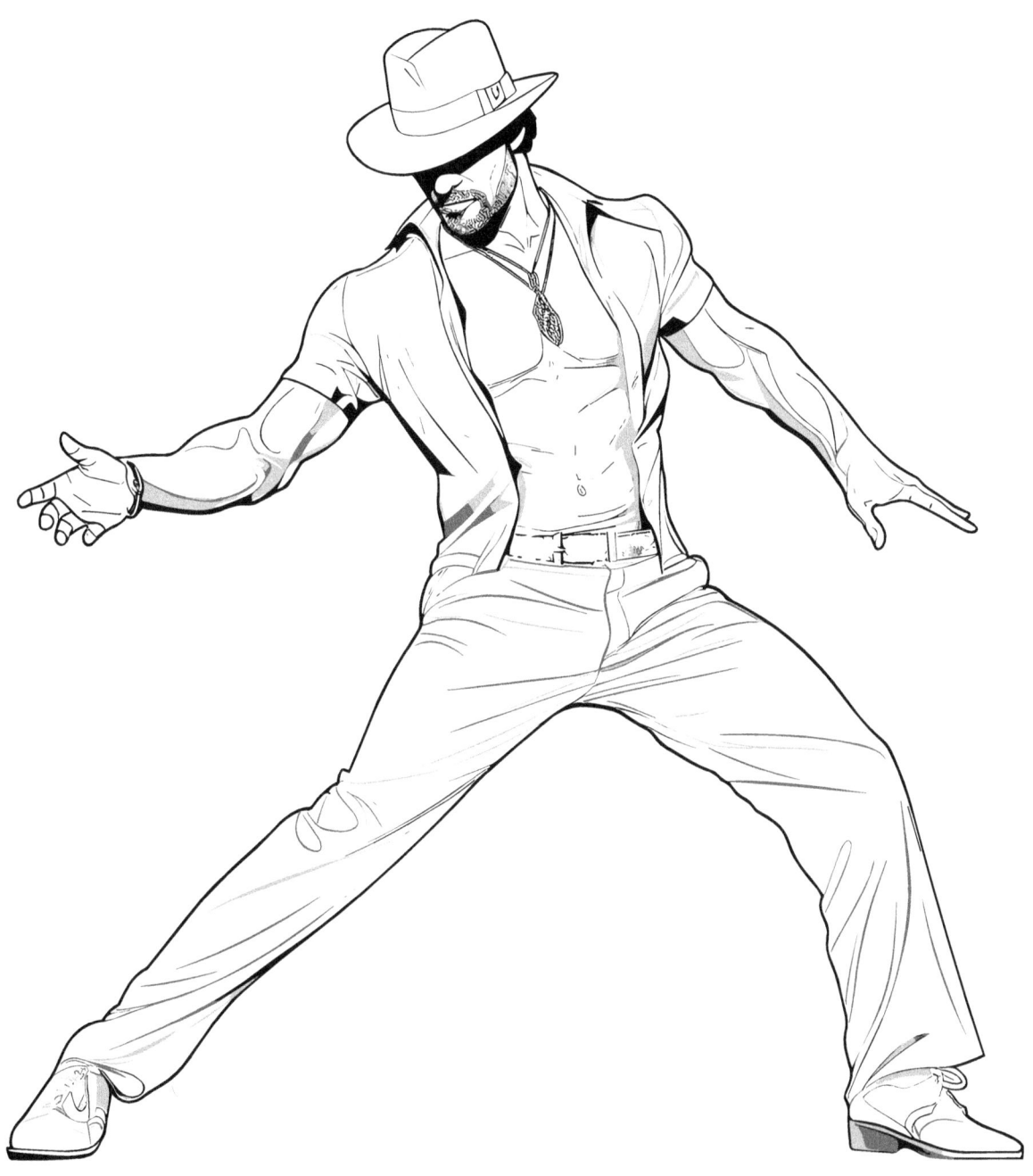

Blank by Design

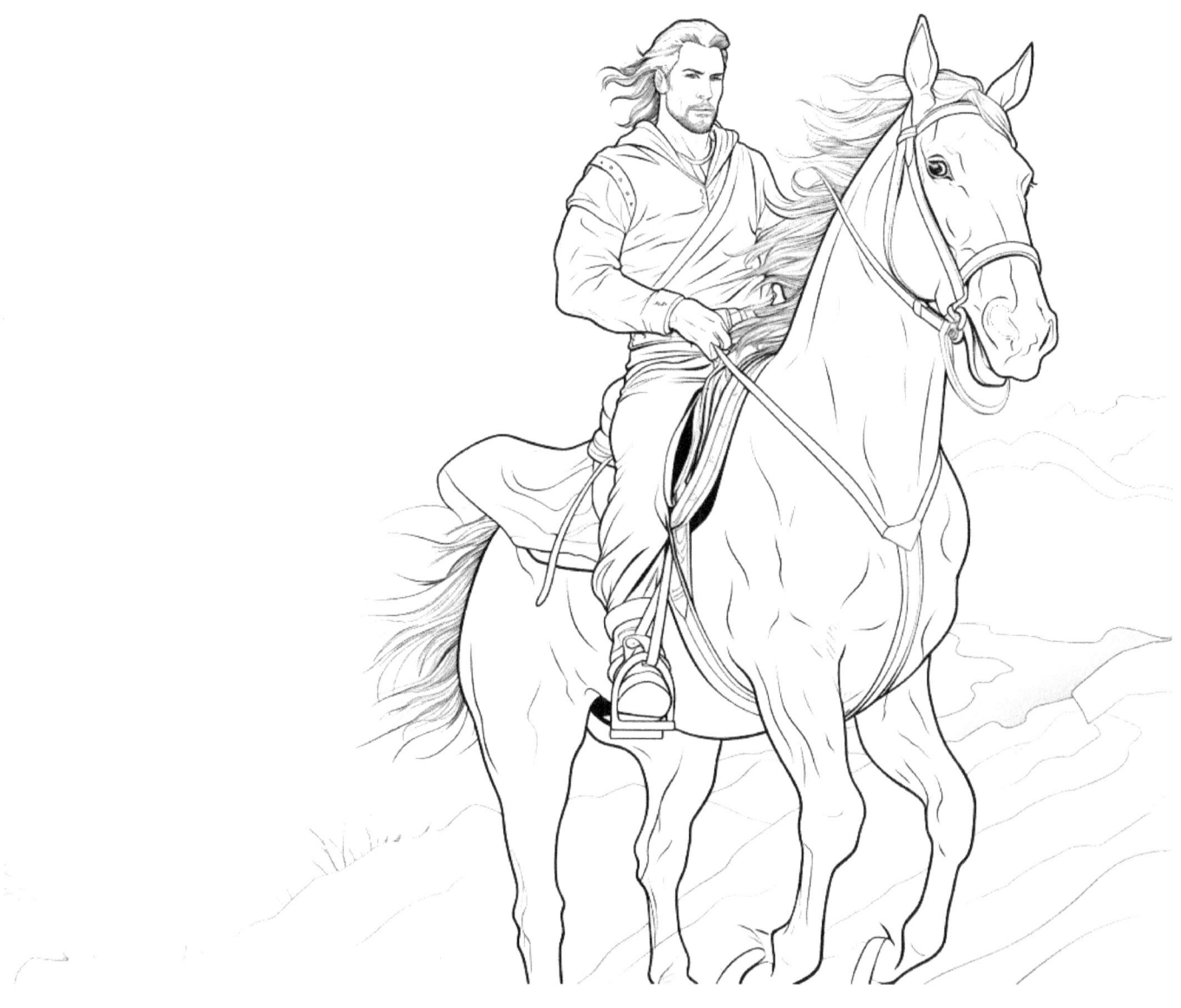

Blank by Design

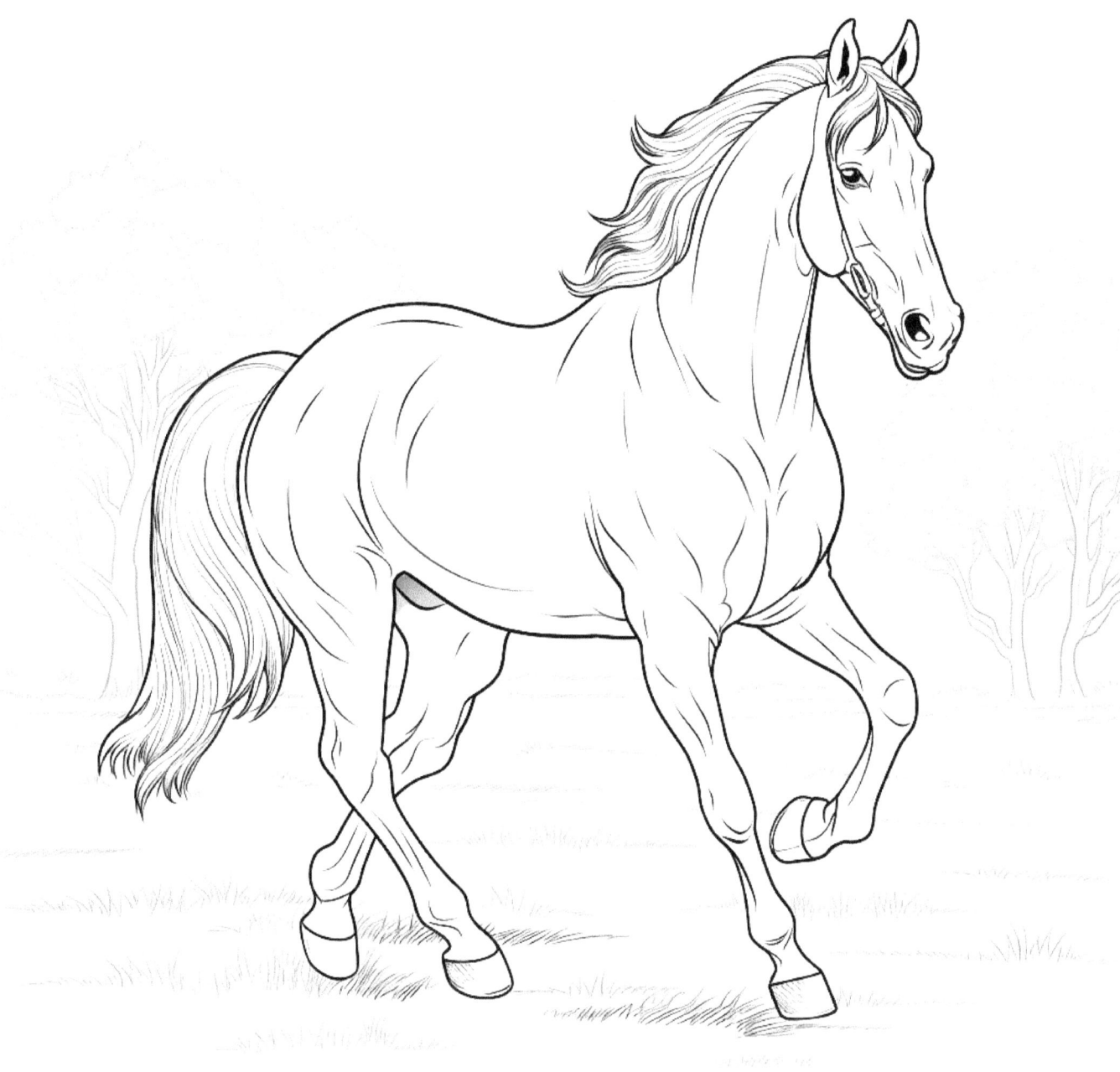

Blank by Design

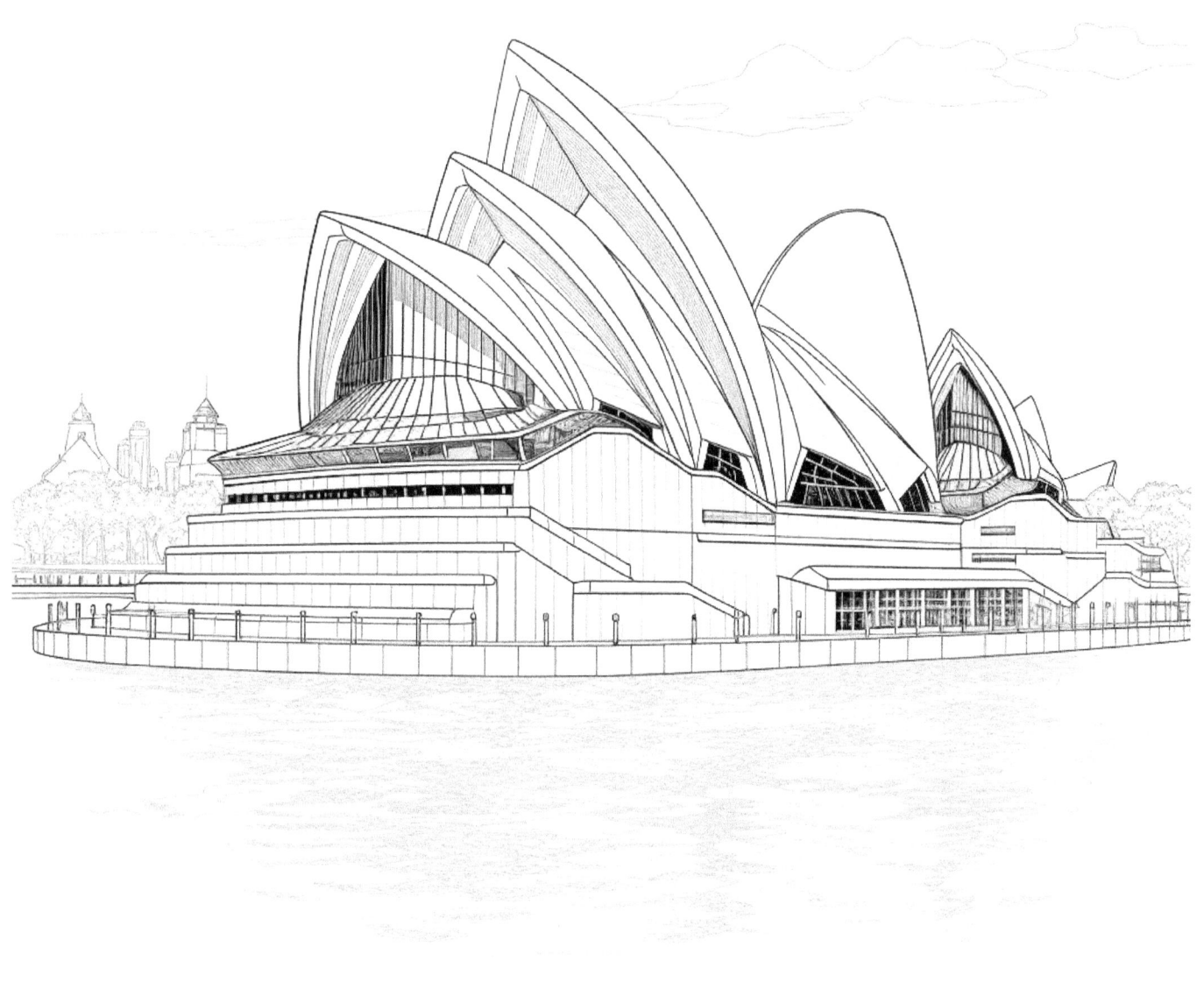

Blank by Design

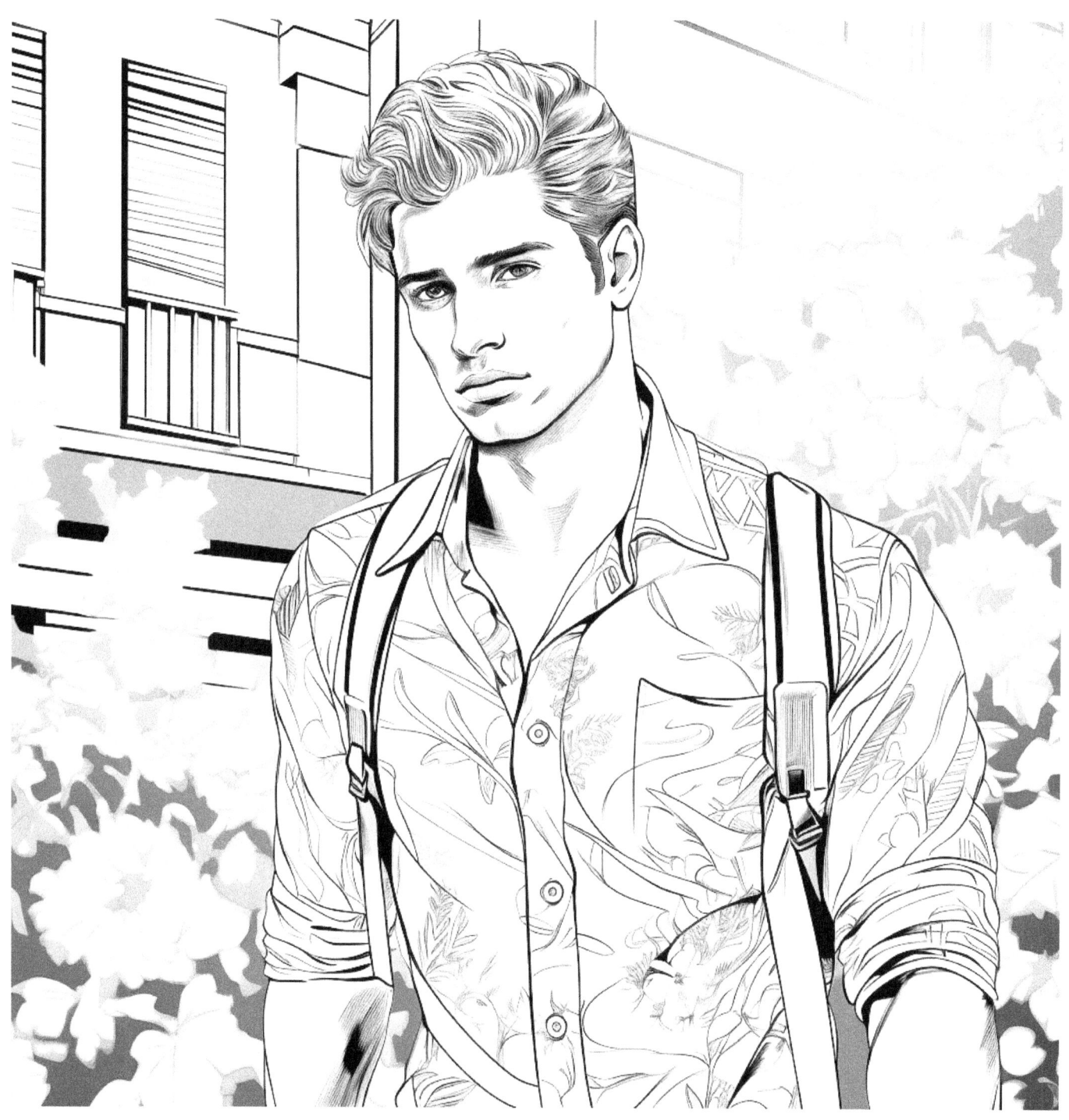

Blank by Design

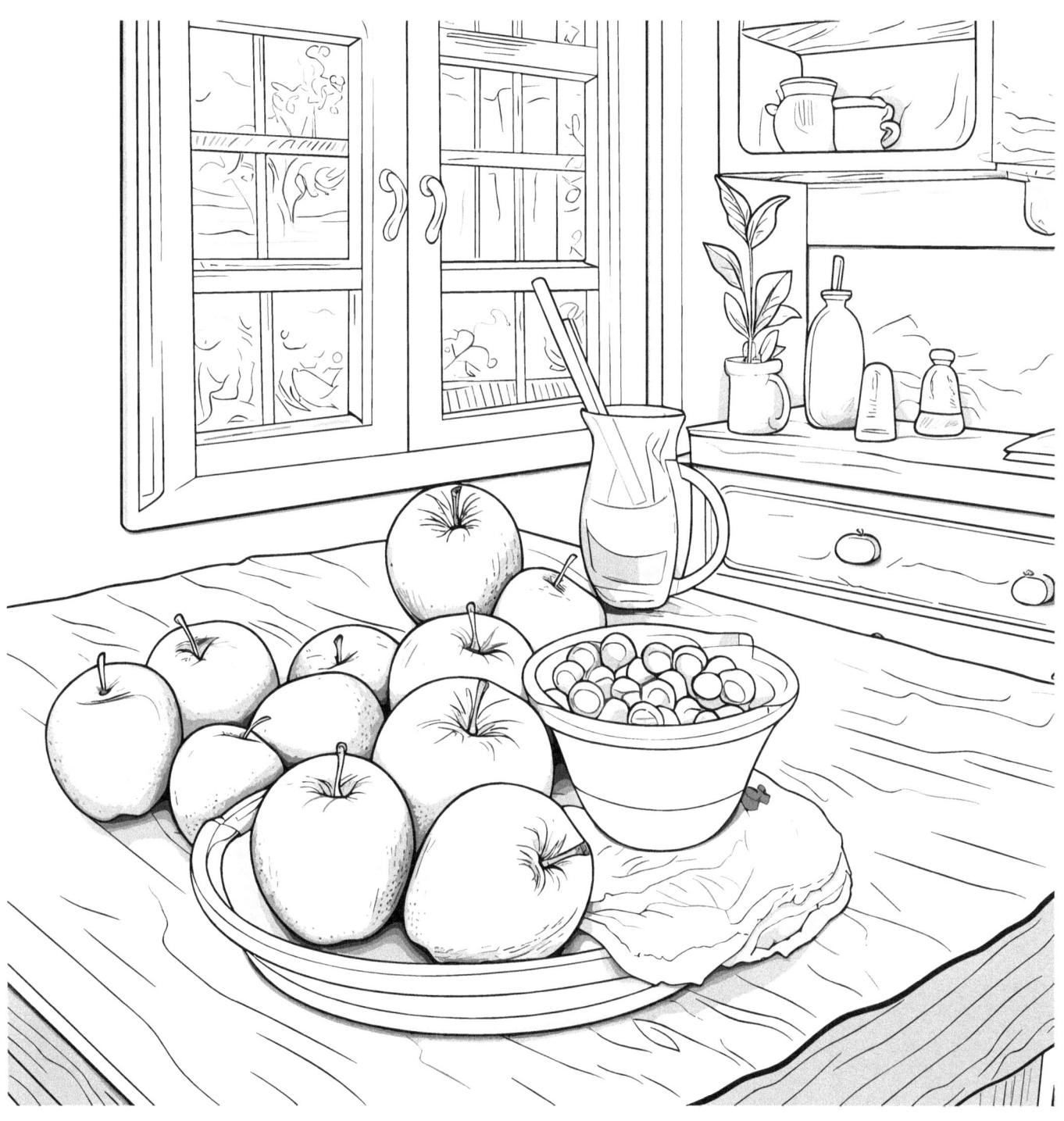

Blank by Design

Balanced Mind Balanced Life

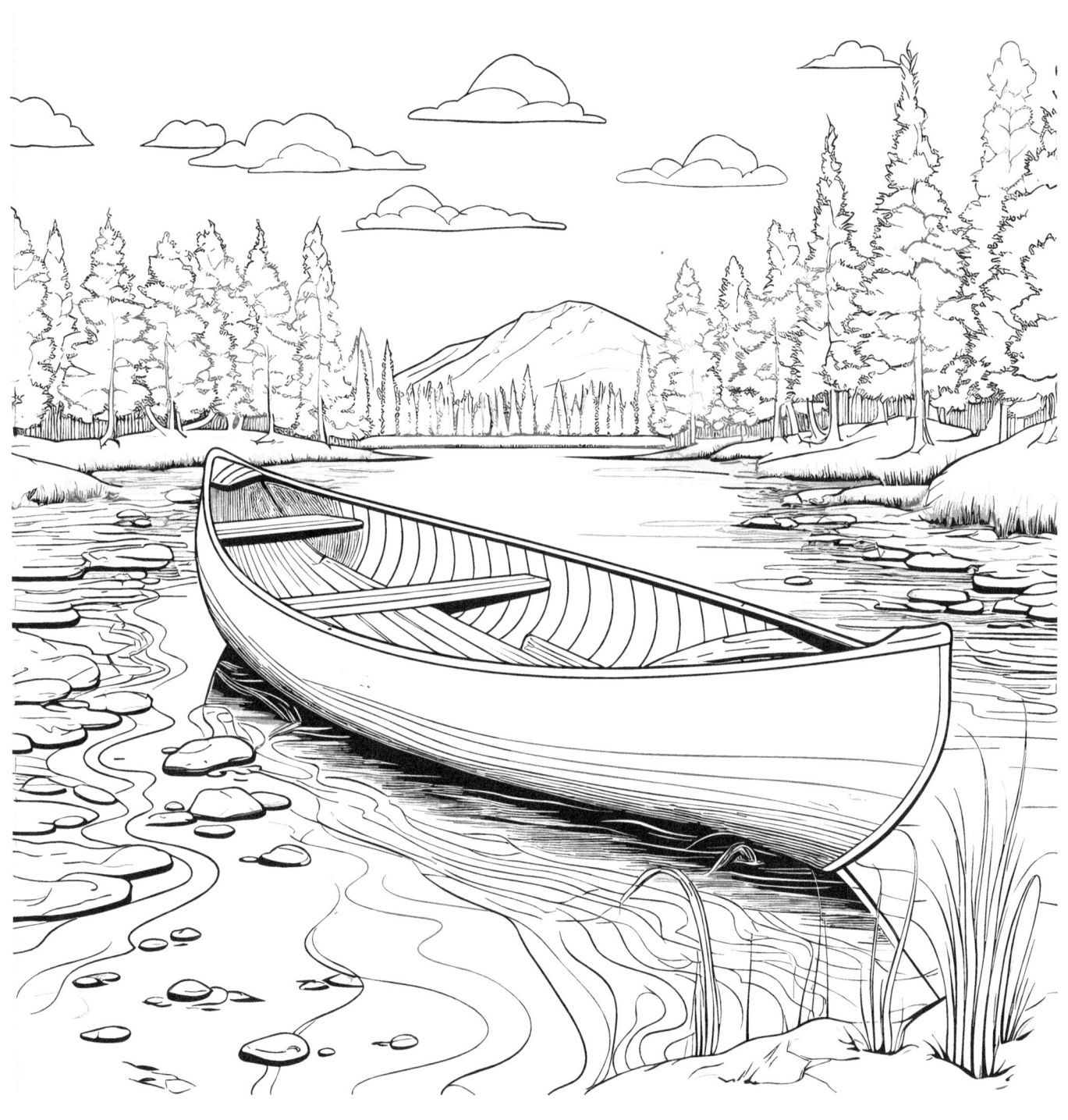

Blank by Design

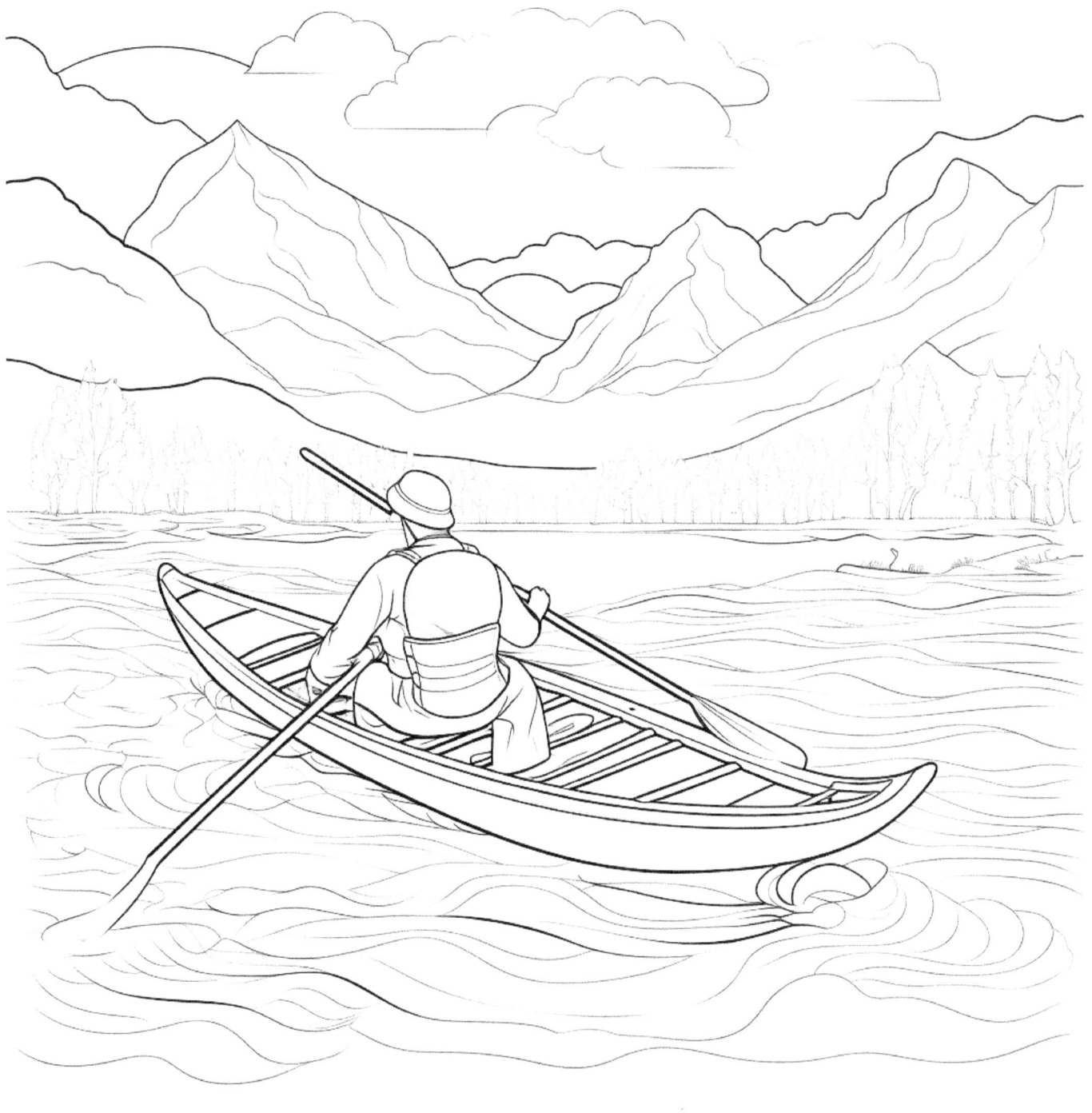

Blank by Design

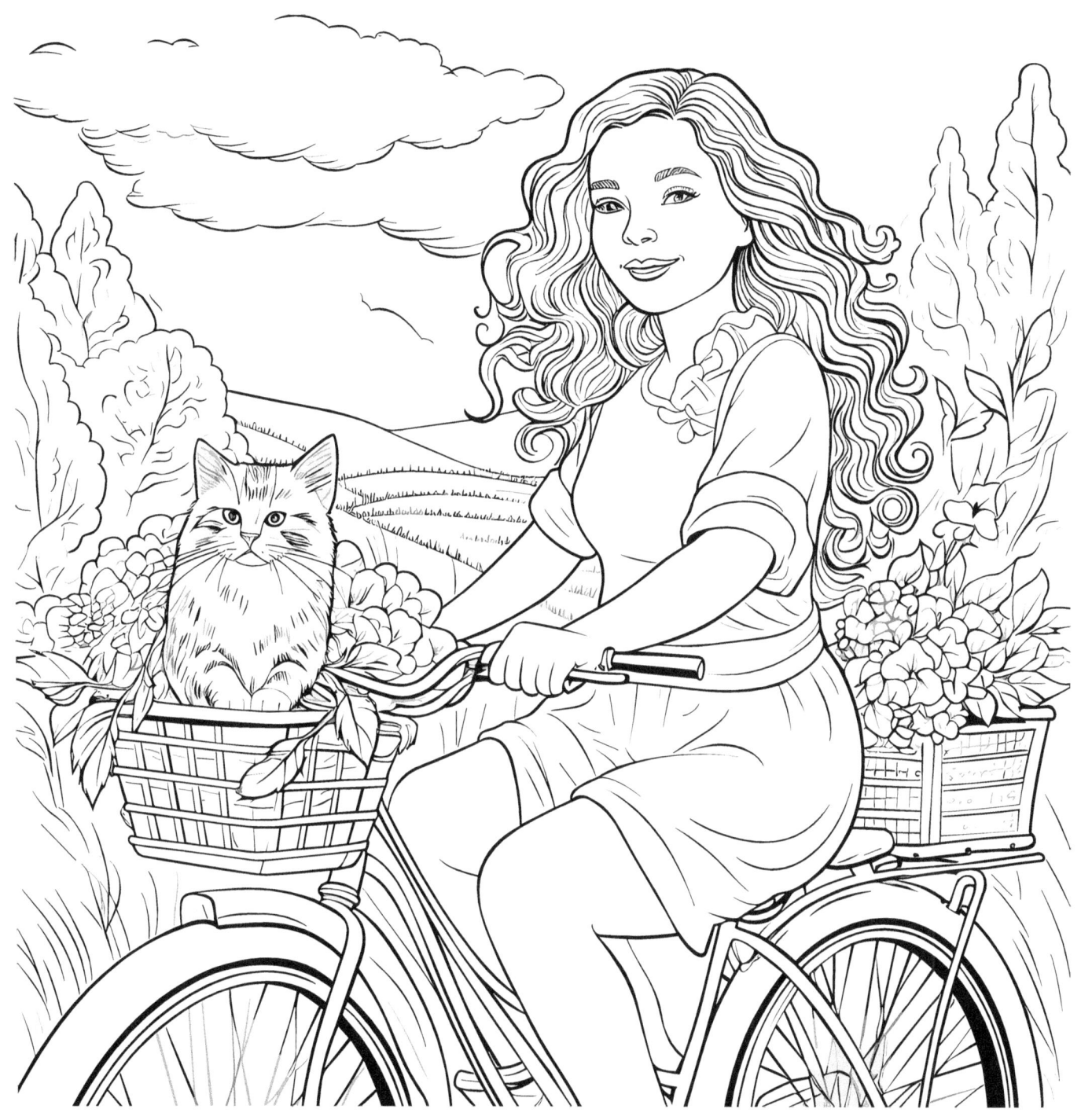

Blank by Design

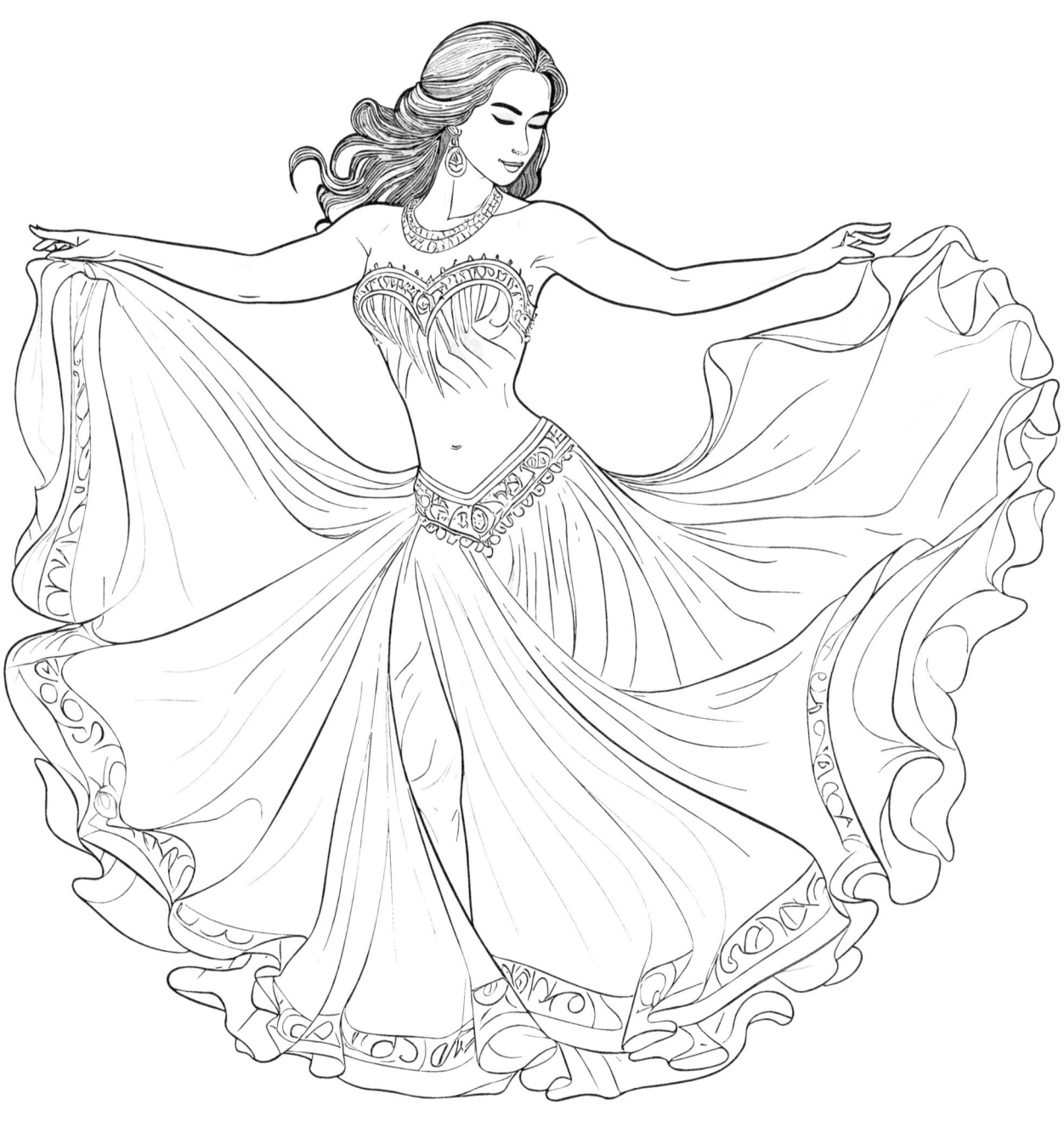

Blank by Design

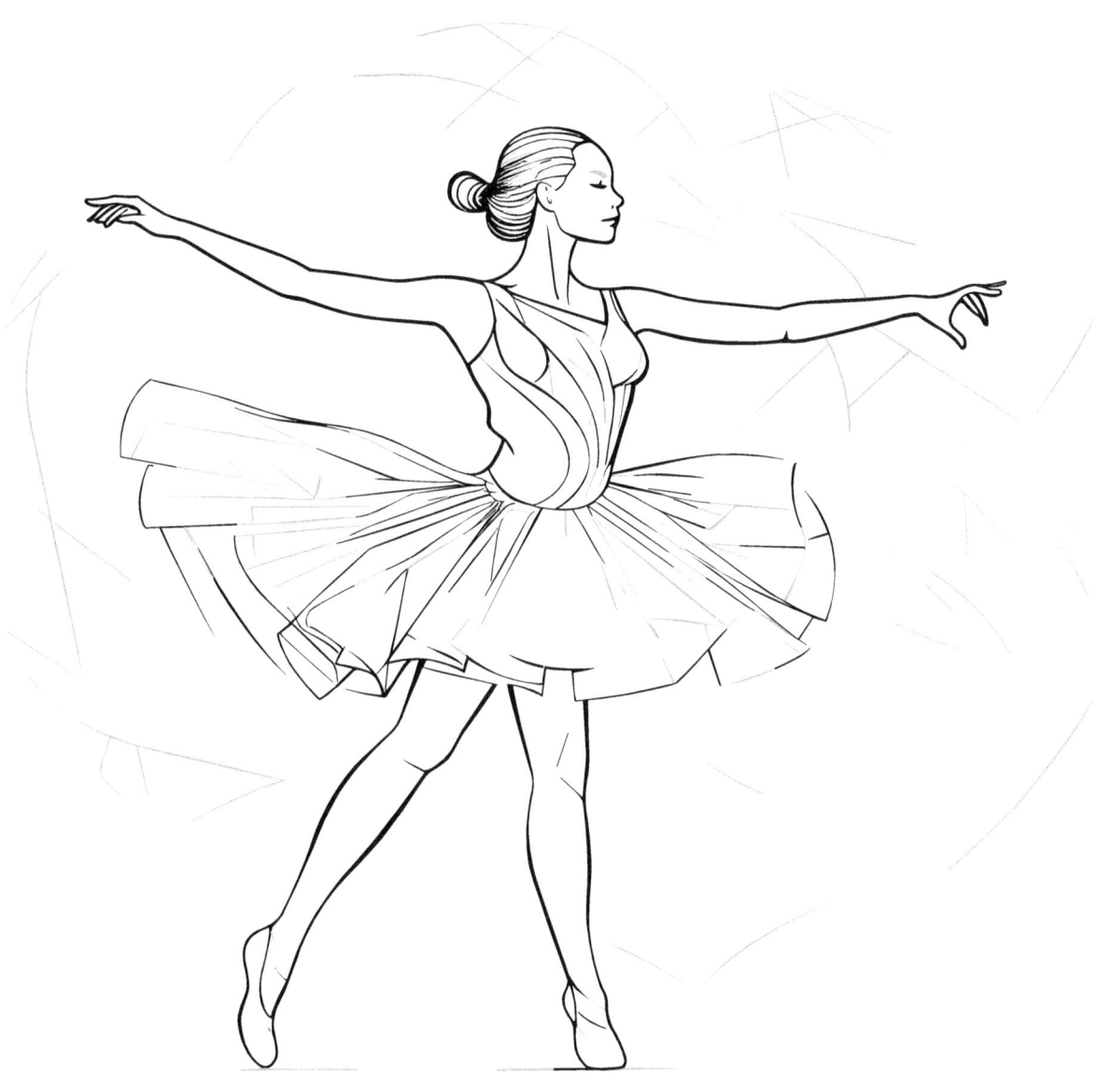

Blank by Design

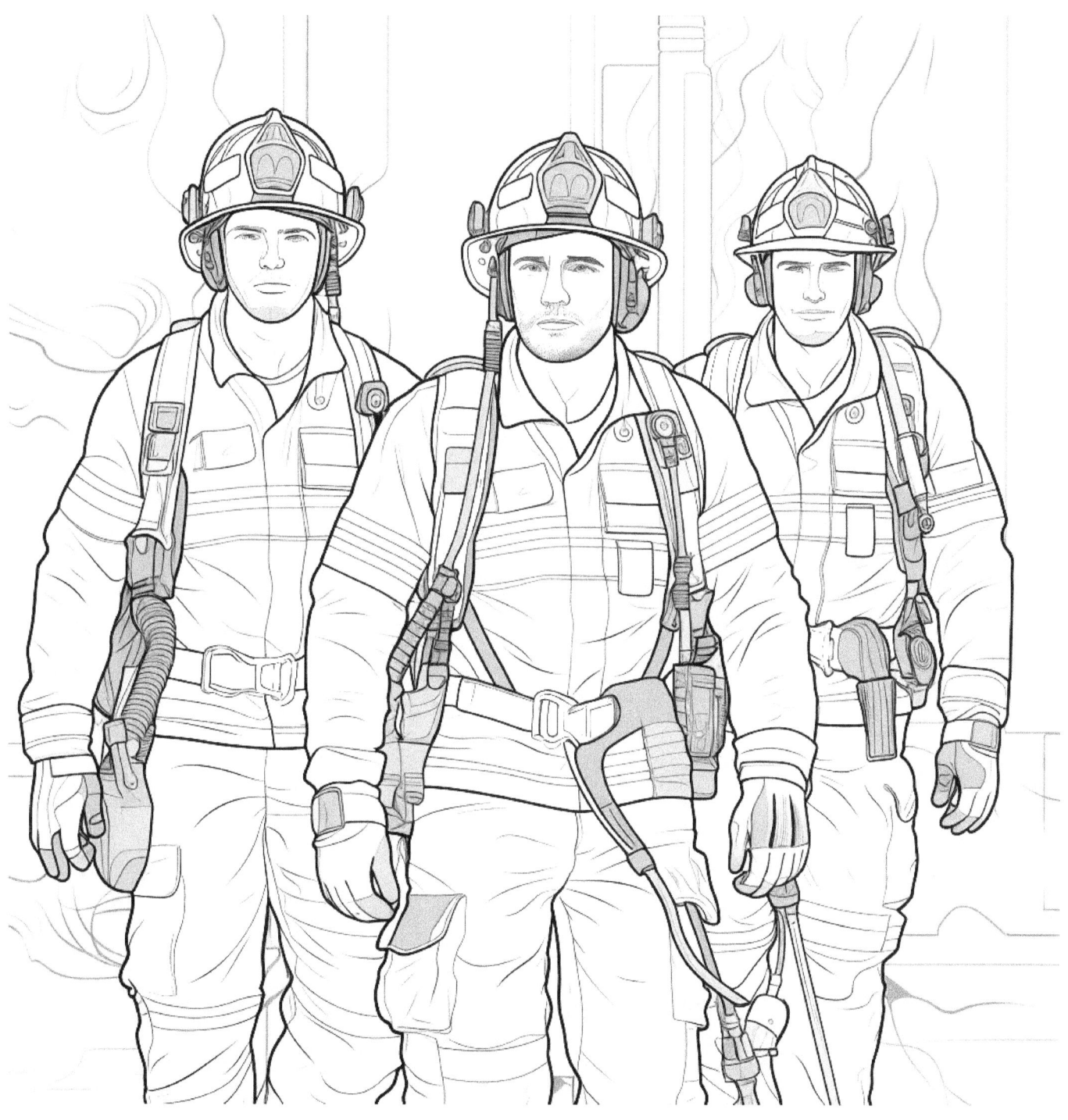

Blank by Design

Balanced Mind Balanced Life

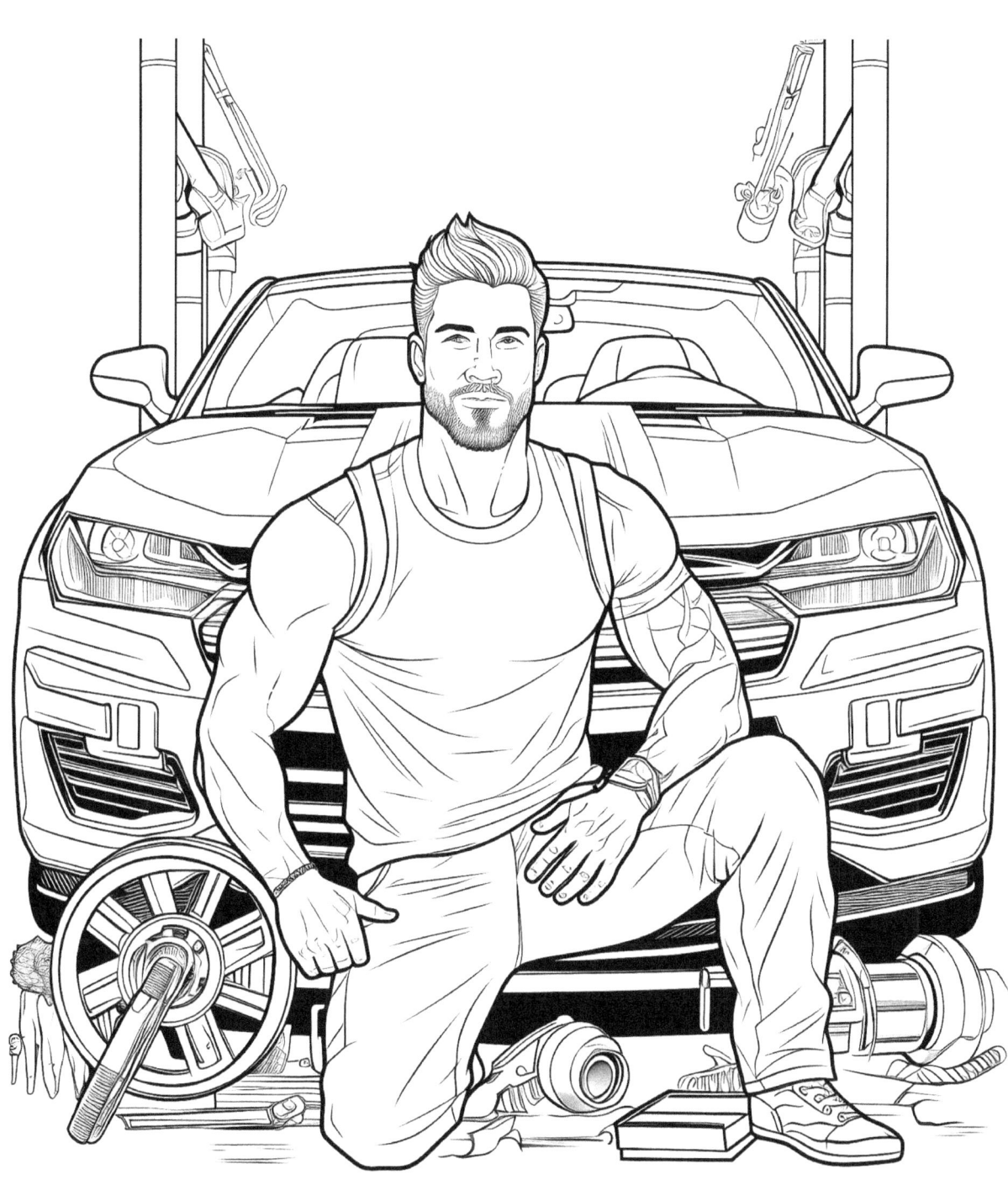

Joe Aguilus

*Blank by
Design*

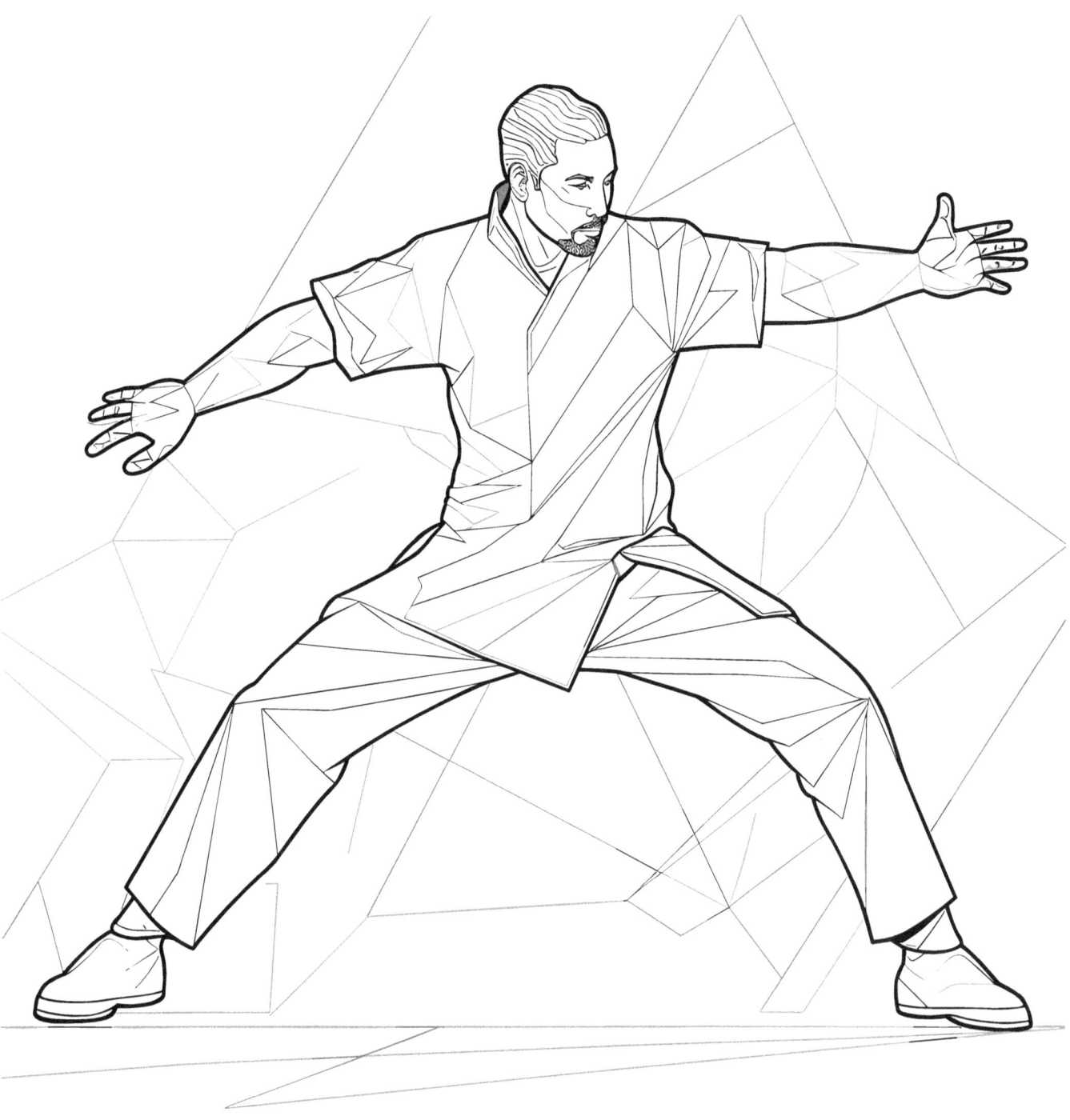

Blank by Design

Balanced Mind Balanced Life

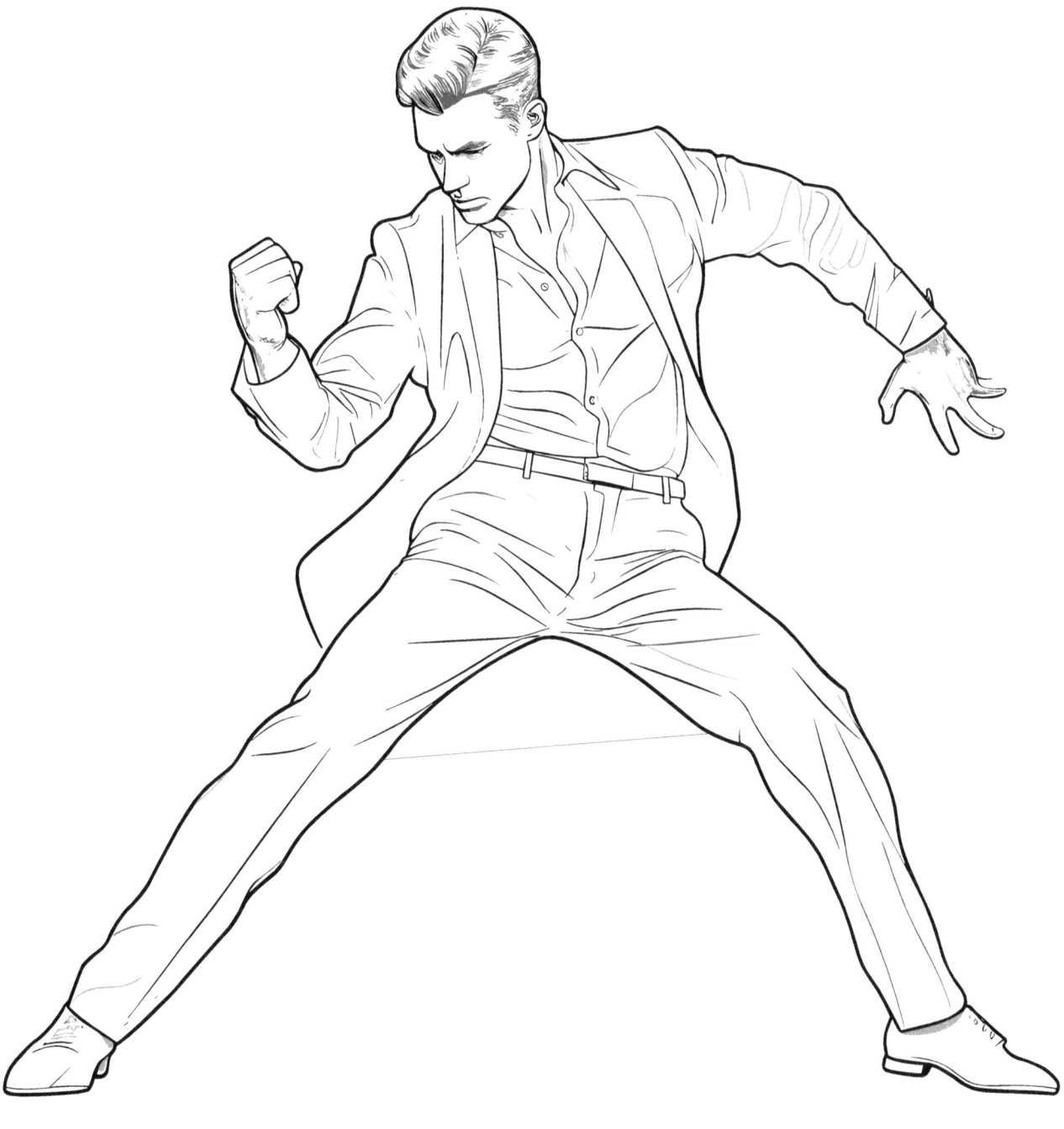

Blank by Design

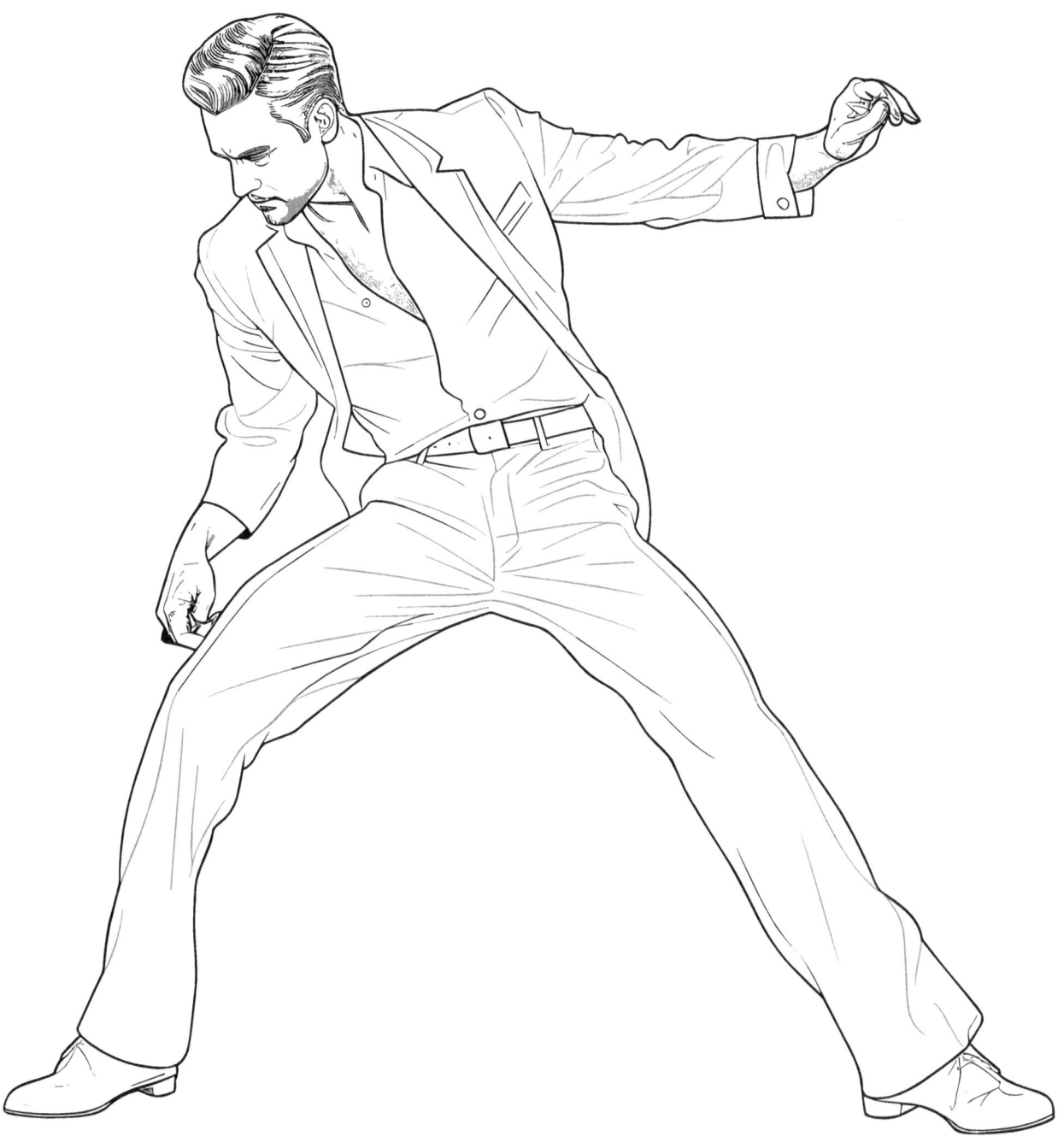

Blank by Design

Balanced Mind Balanced Life

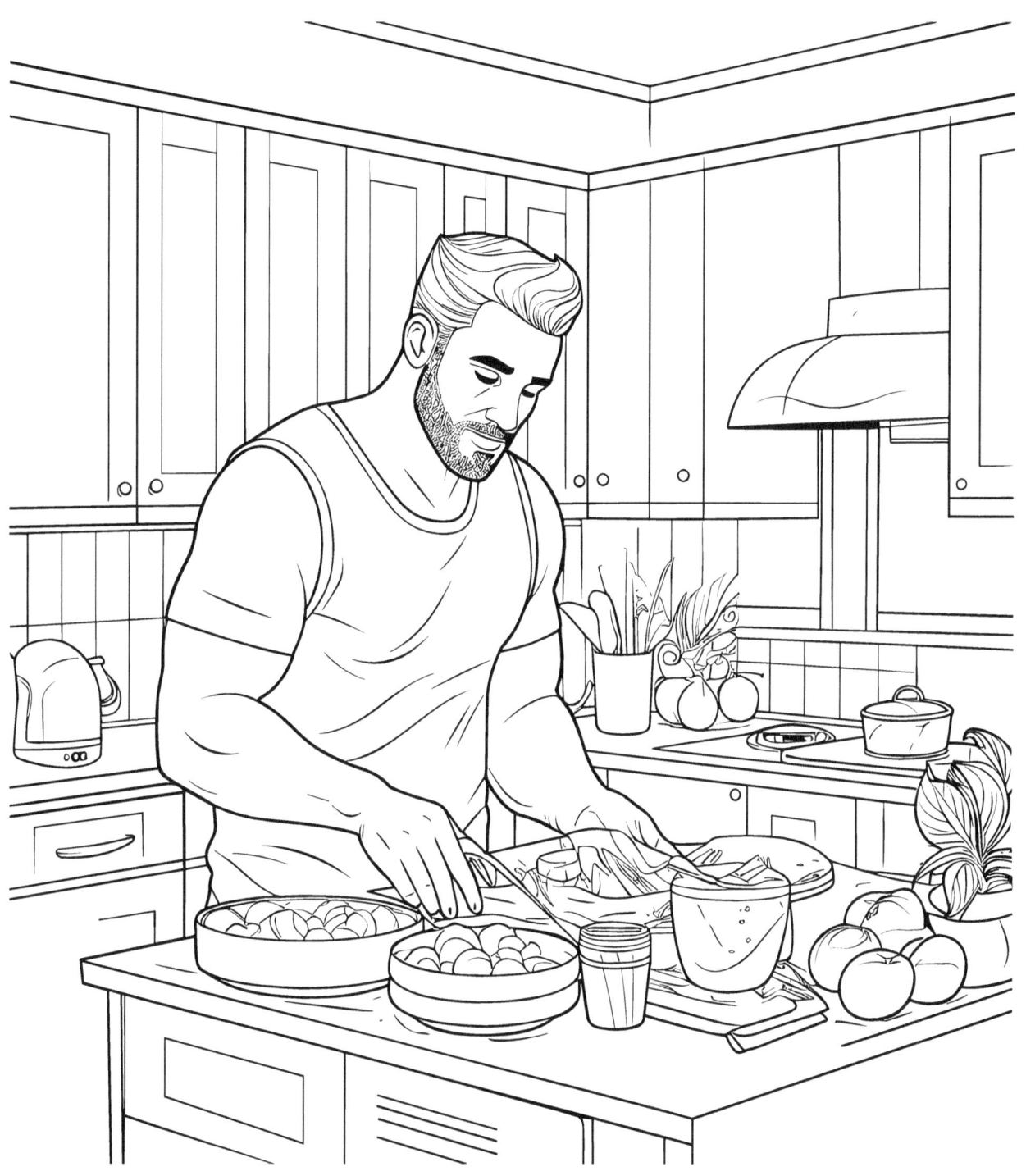

Blank by Design

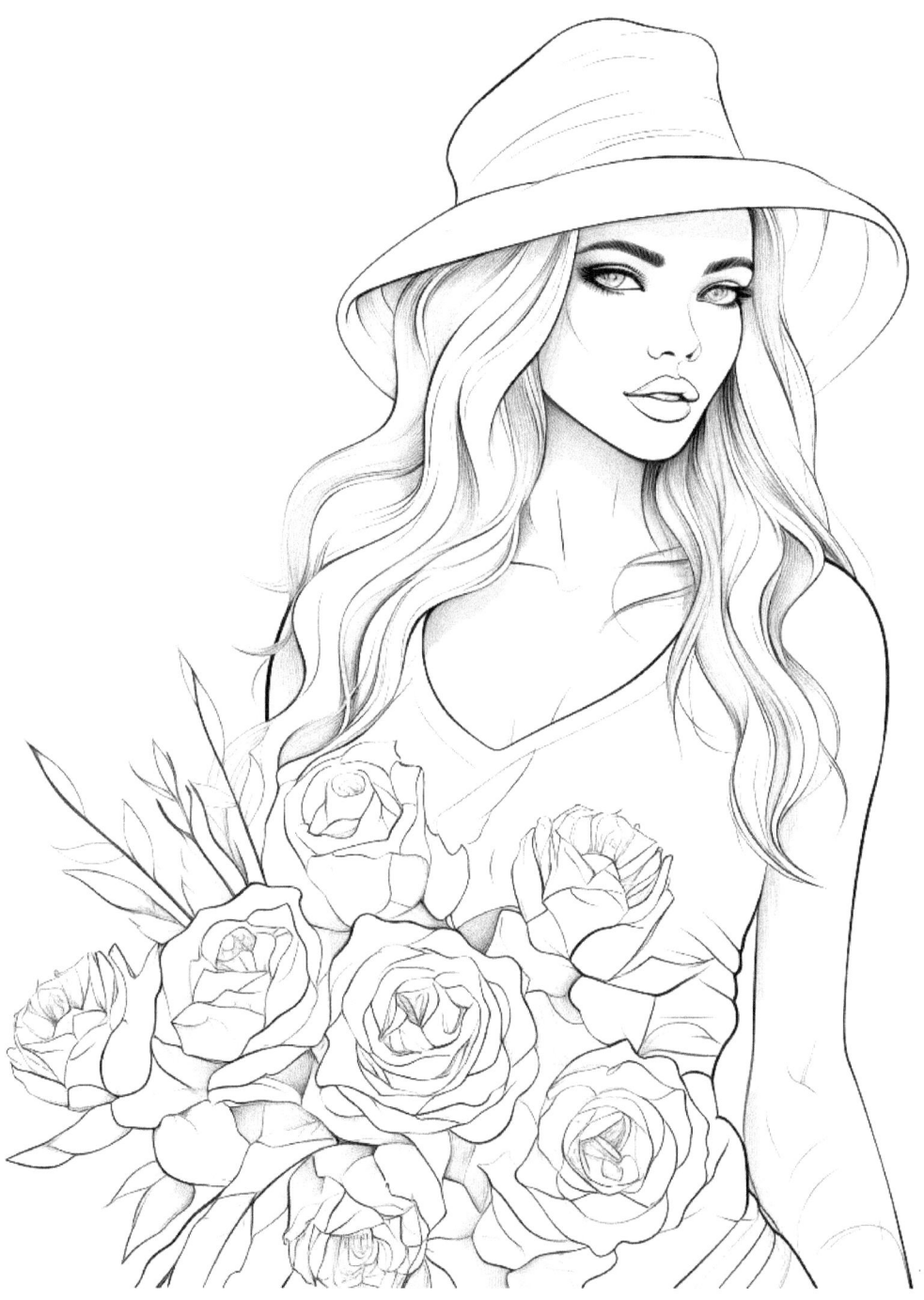

Blank by Design

Balanced Mind Balanced Life

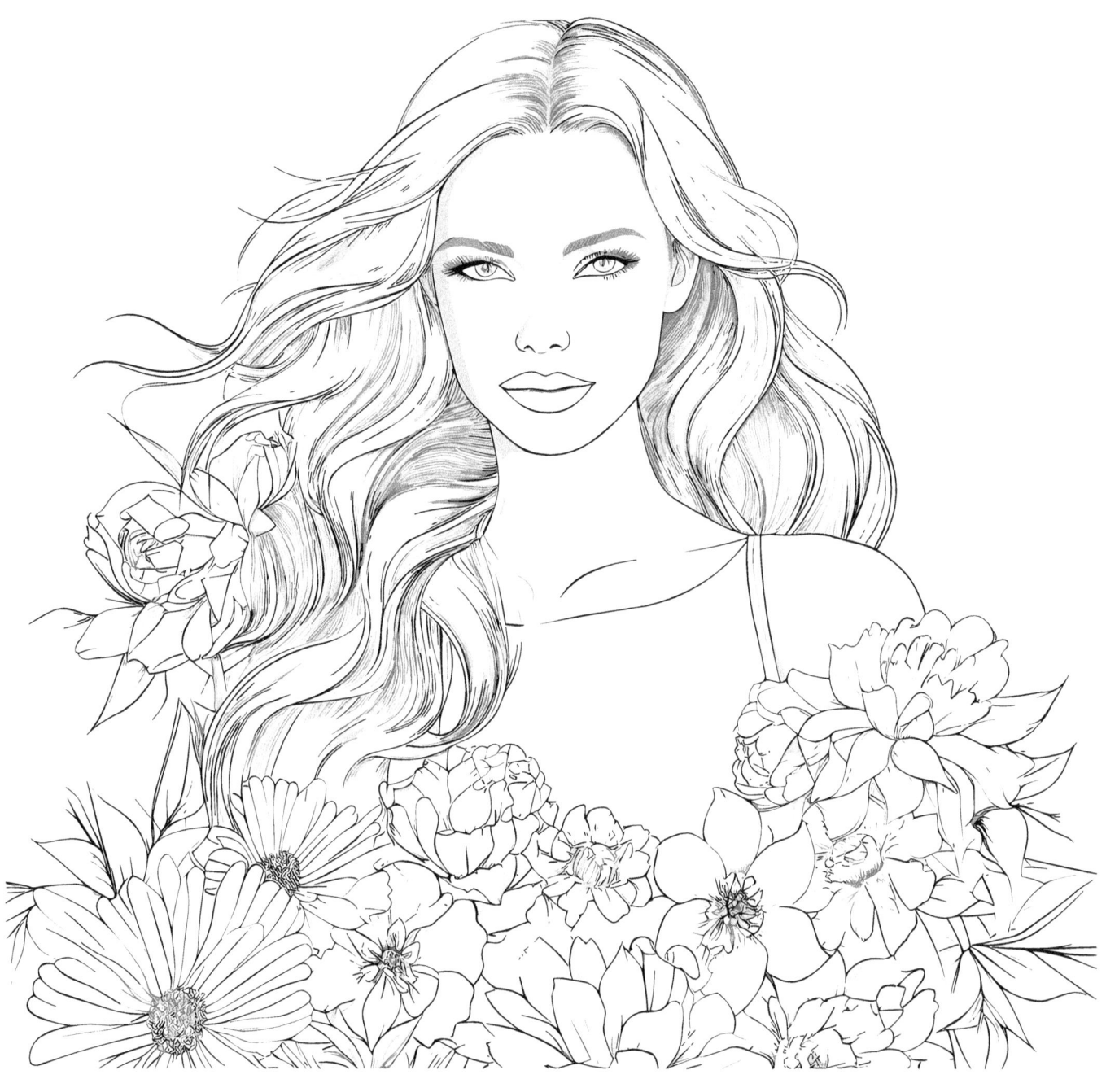

Blank by Design

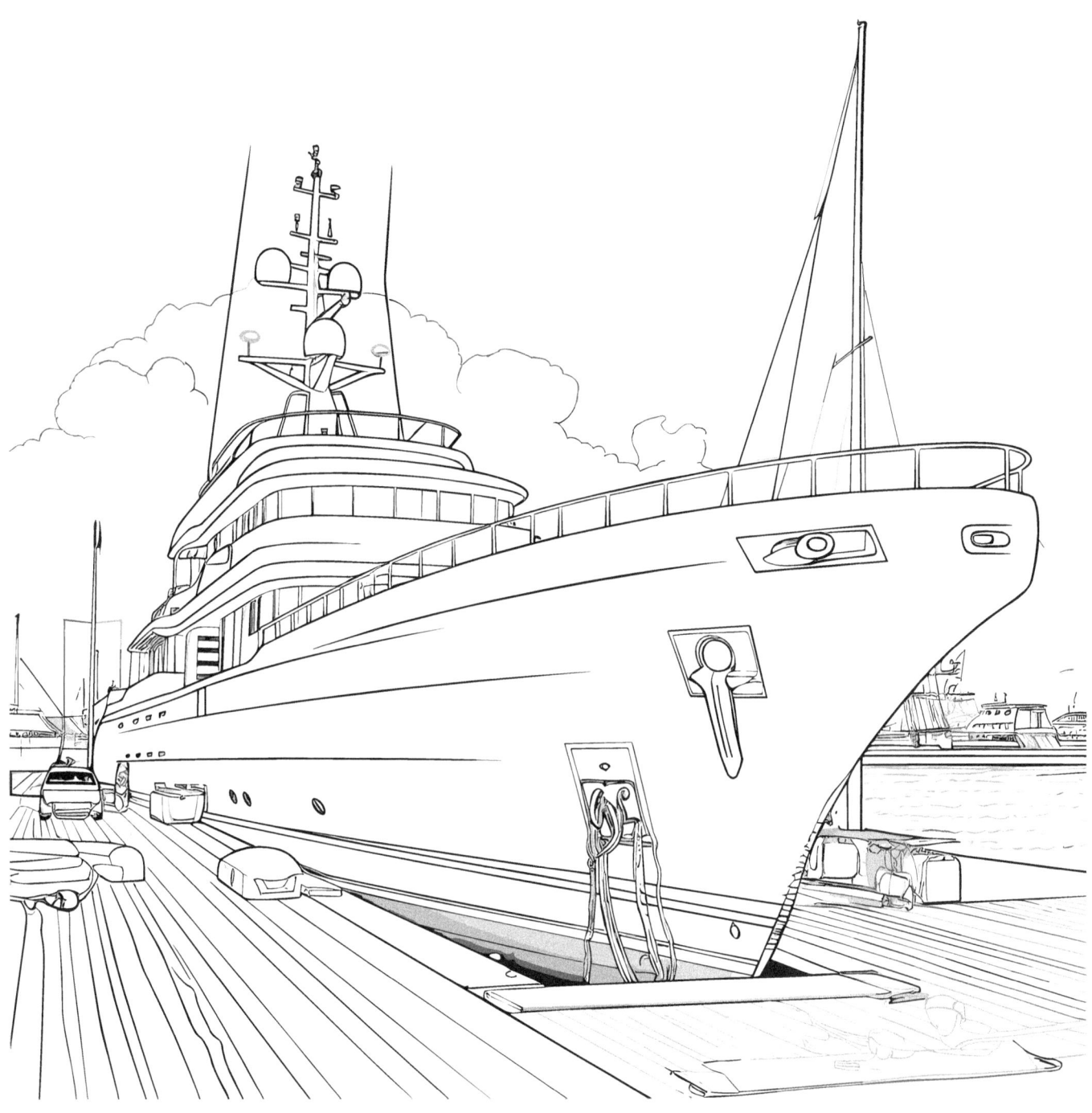

Blank by Design

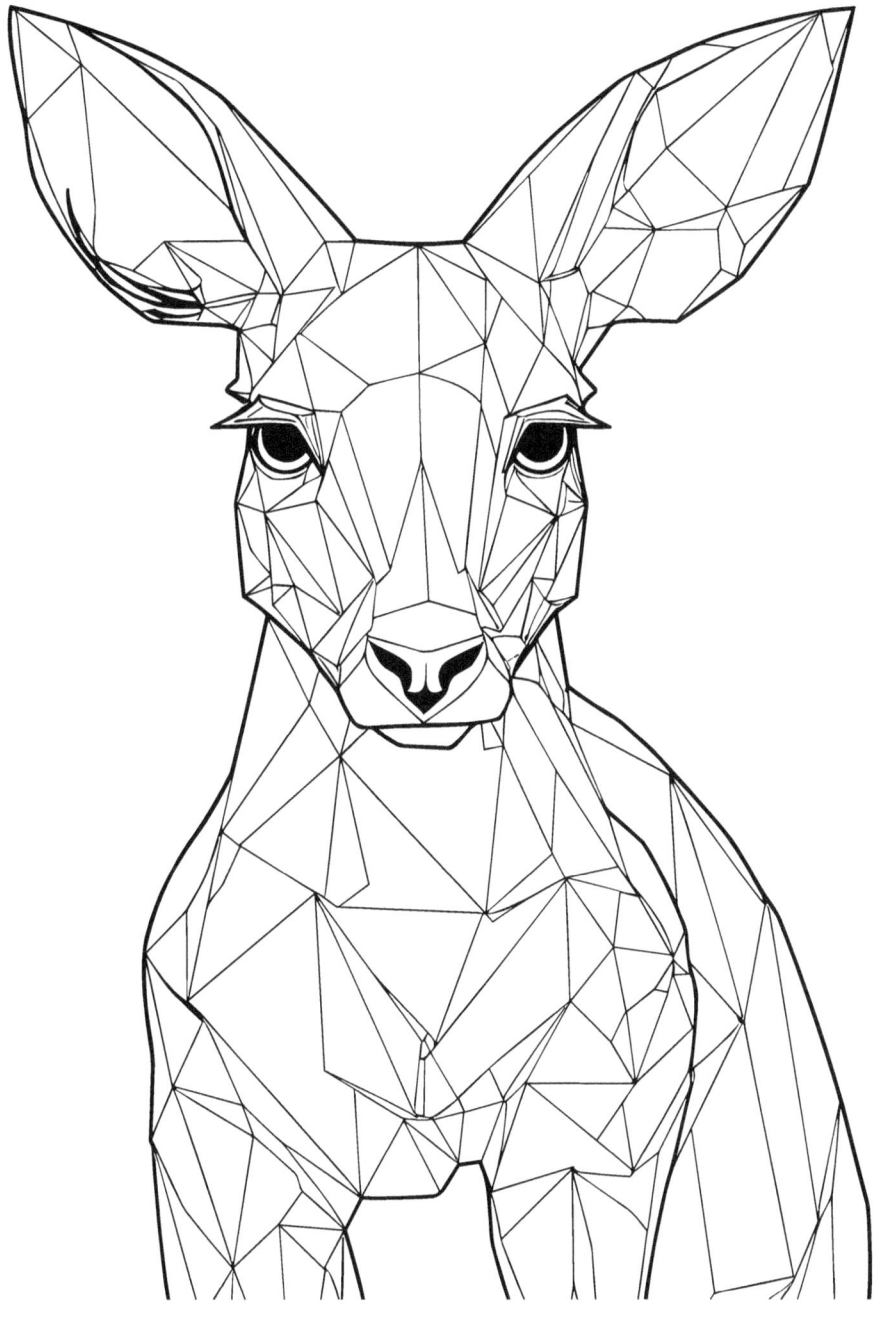

Joe Aguilus

Blank by
Design

Balanced Mind Balanced Life

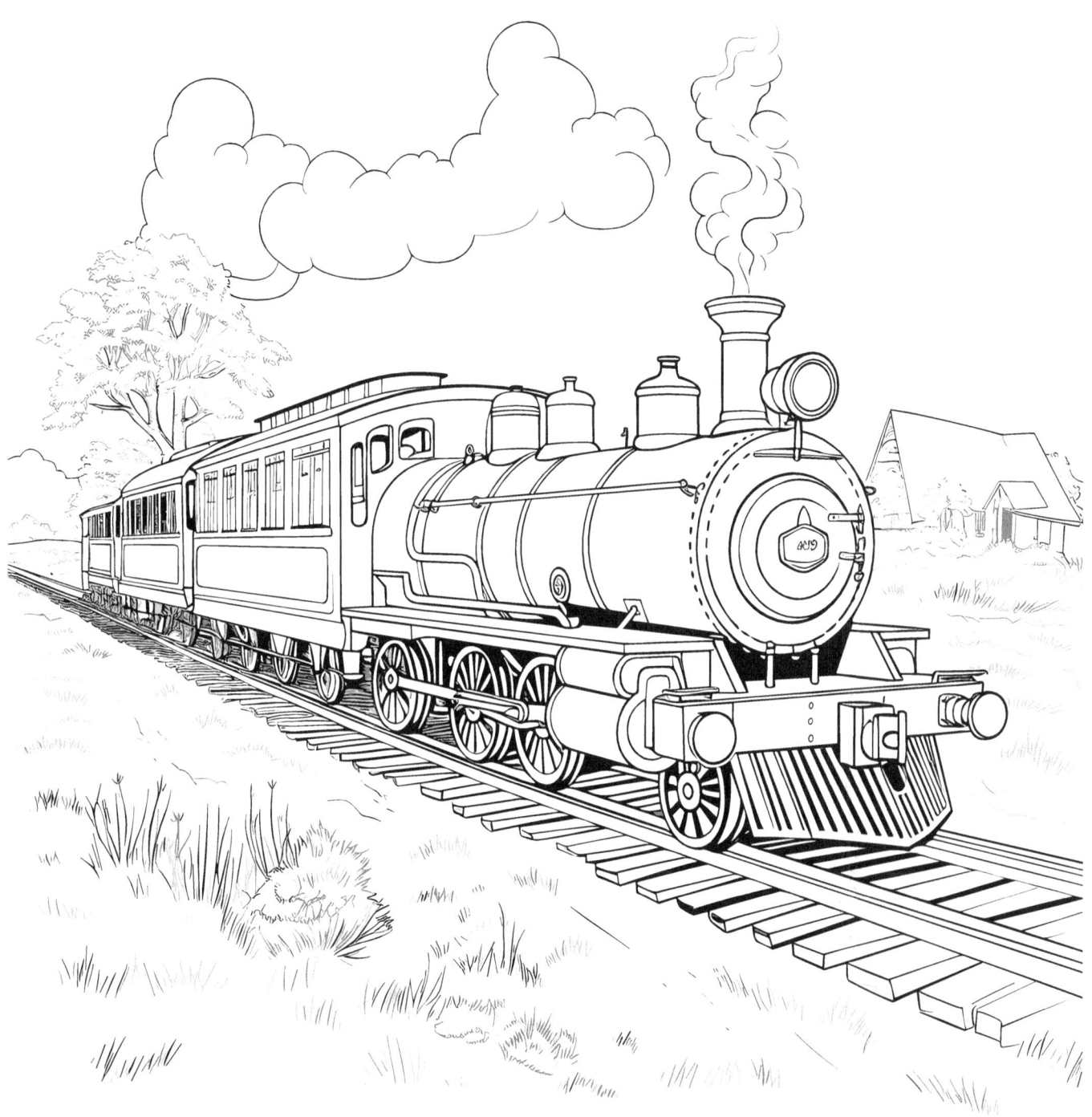

Blank by Design

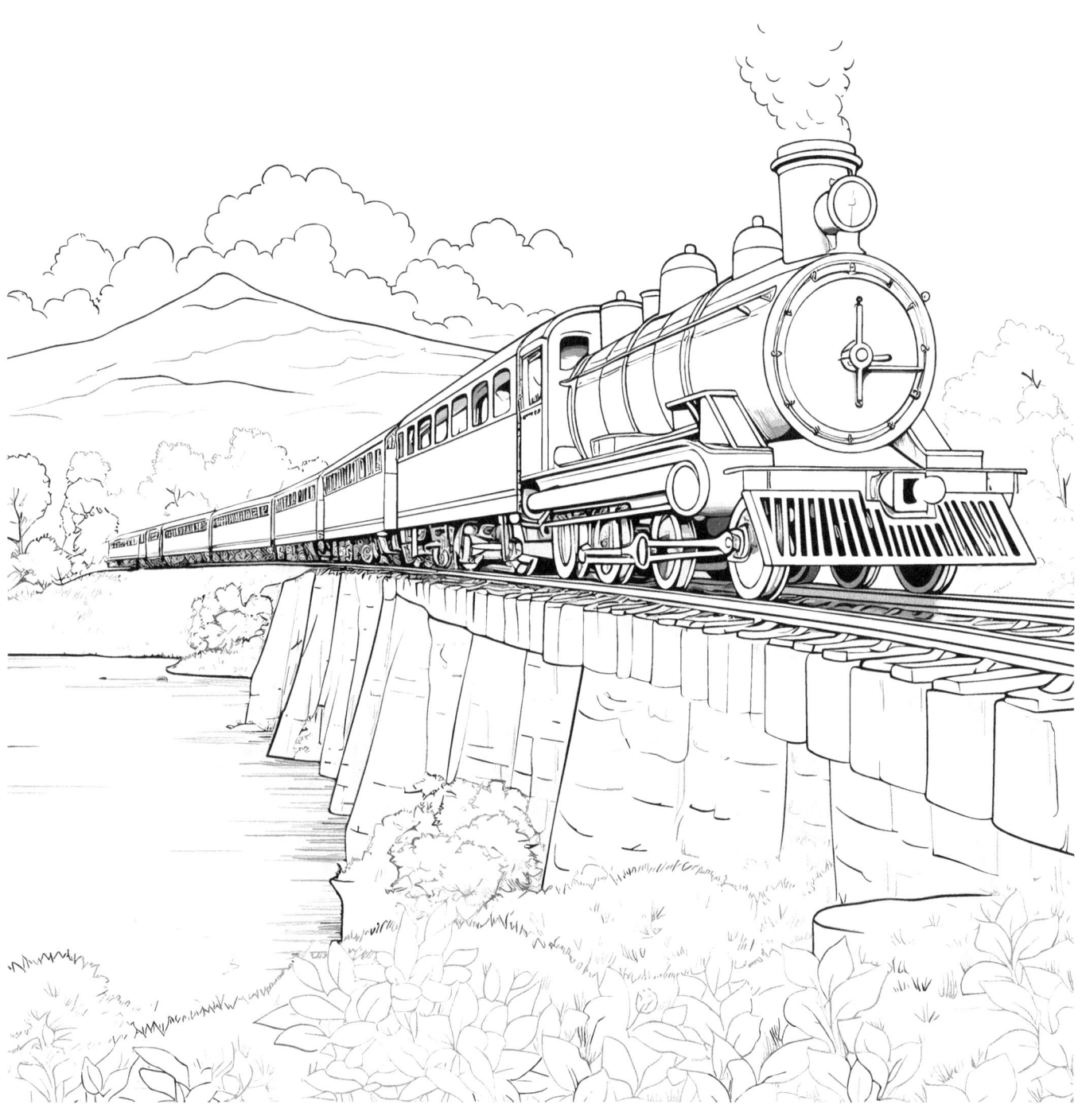

Blank by Design

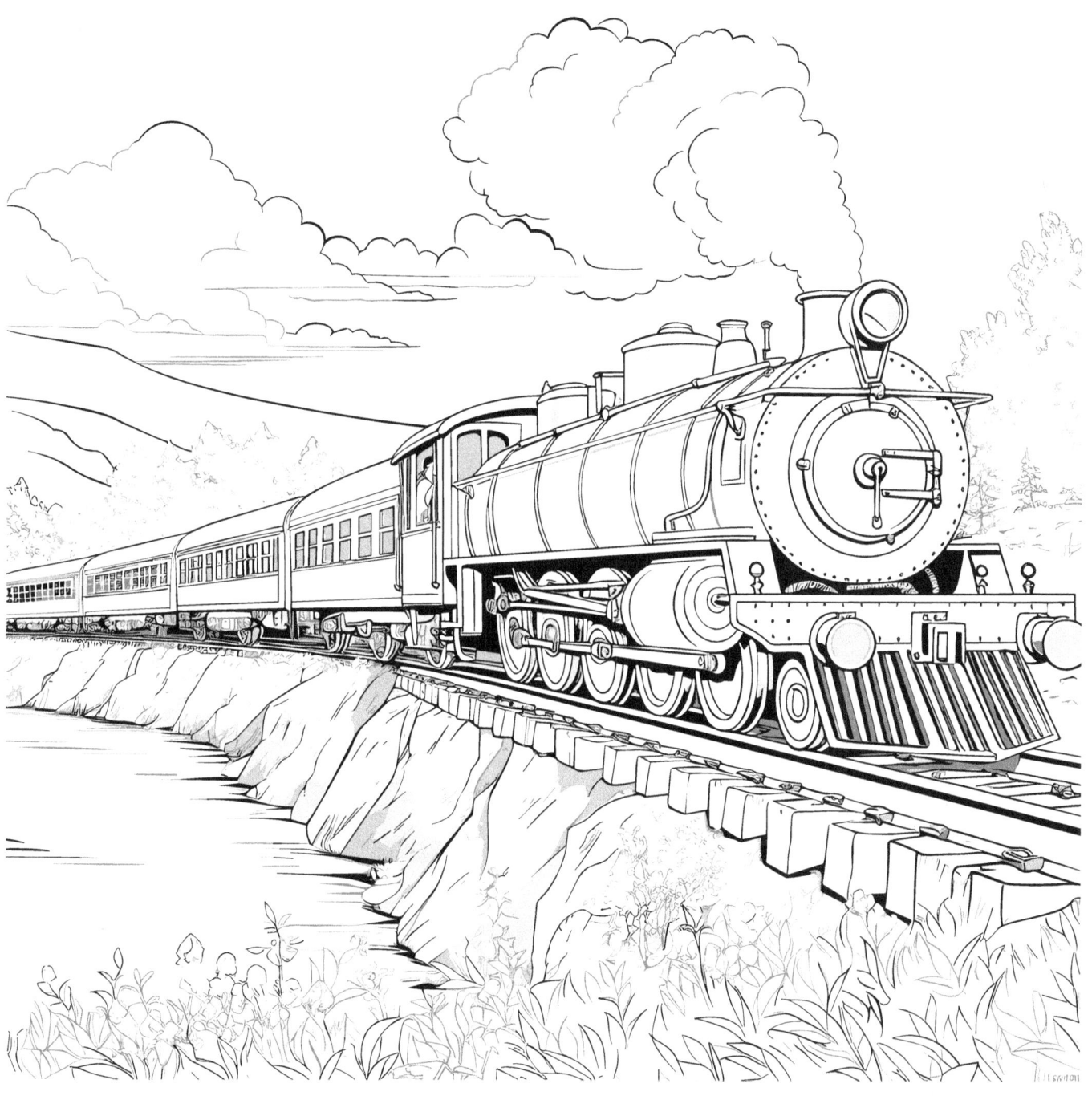

Blank by Design

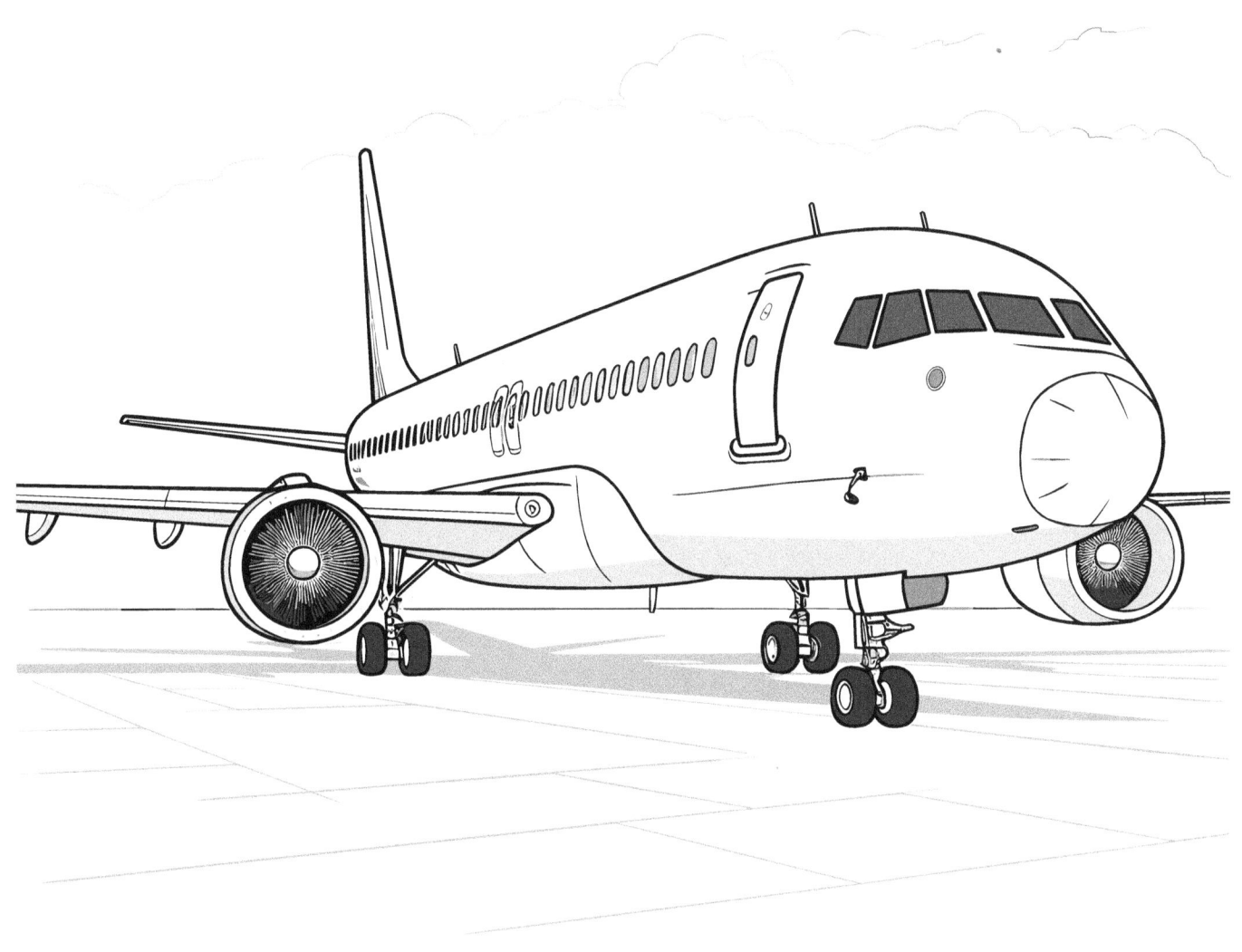

Blank by Design

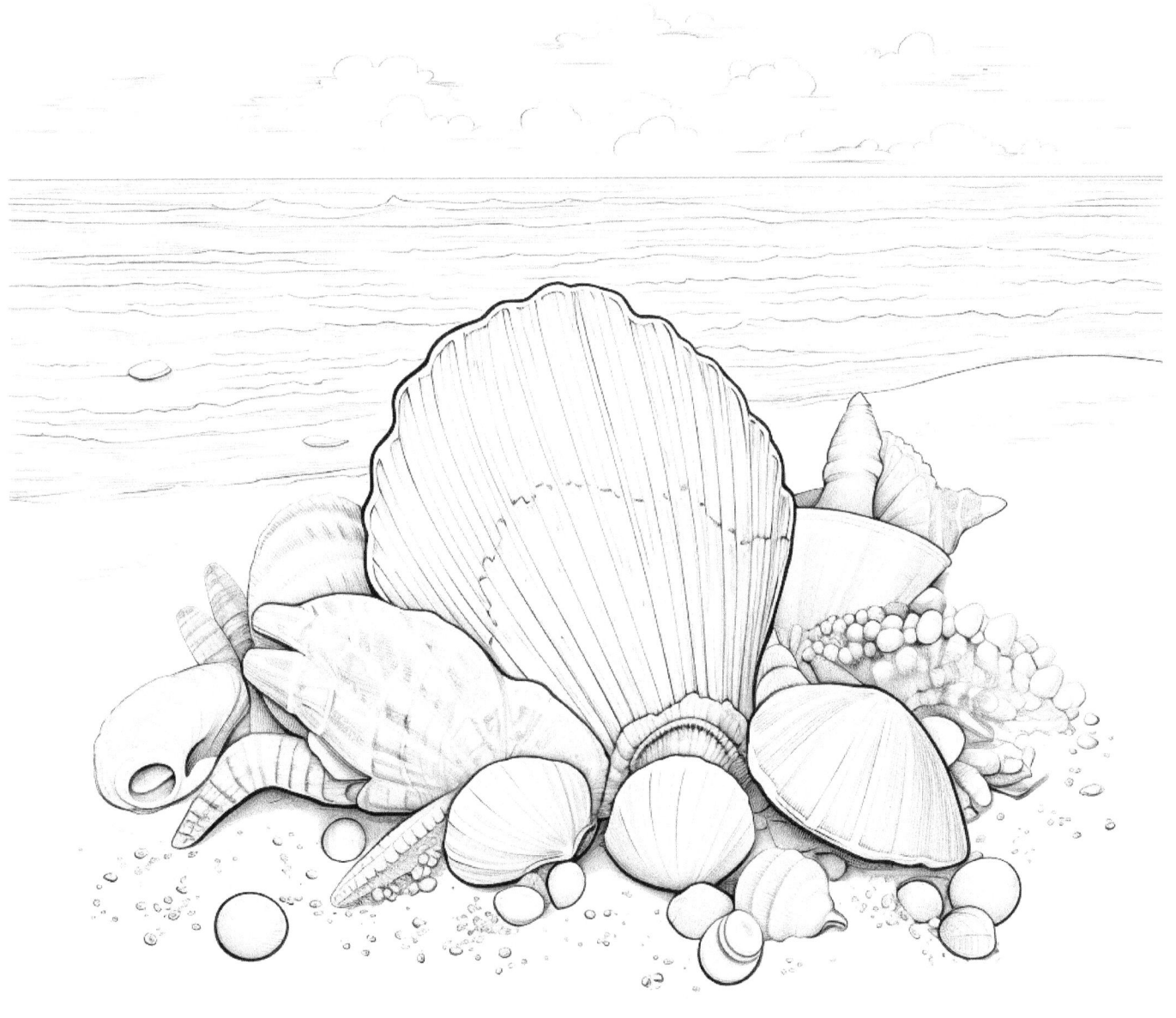

Blank by Design

Balanced Mind Balanced Life

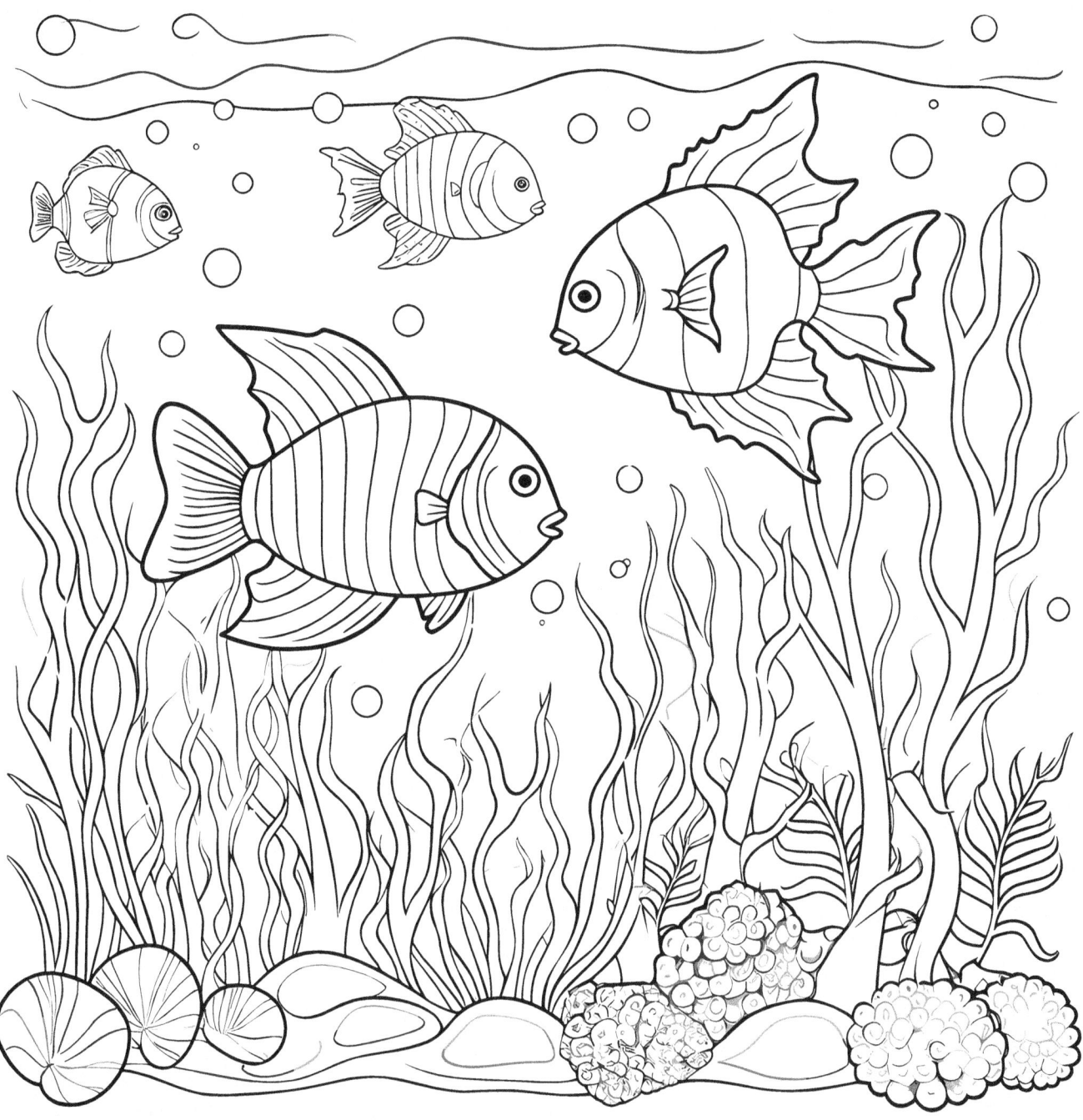

Blank by Design

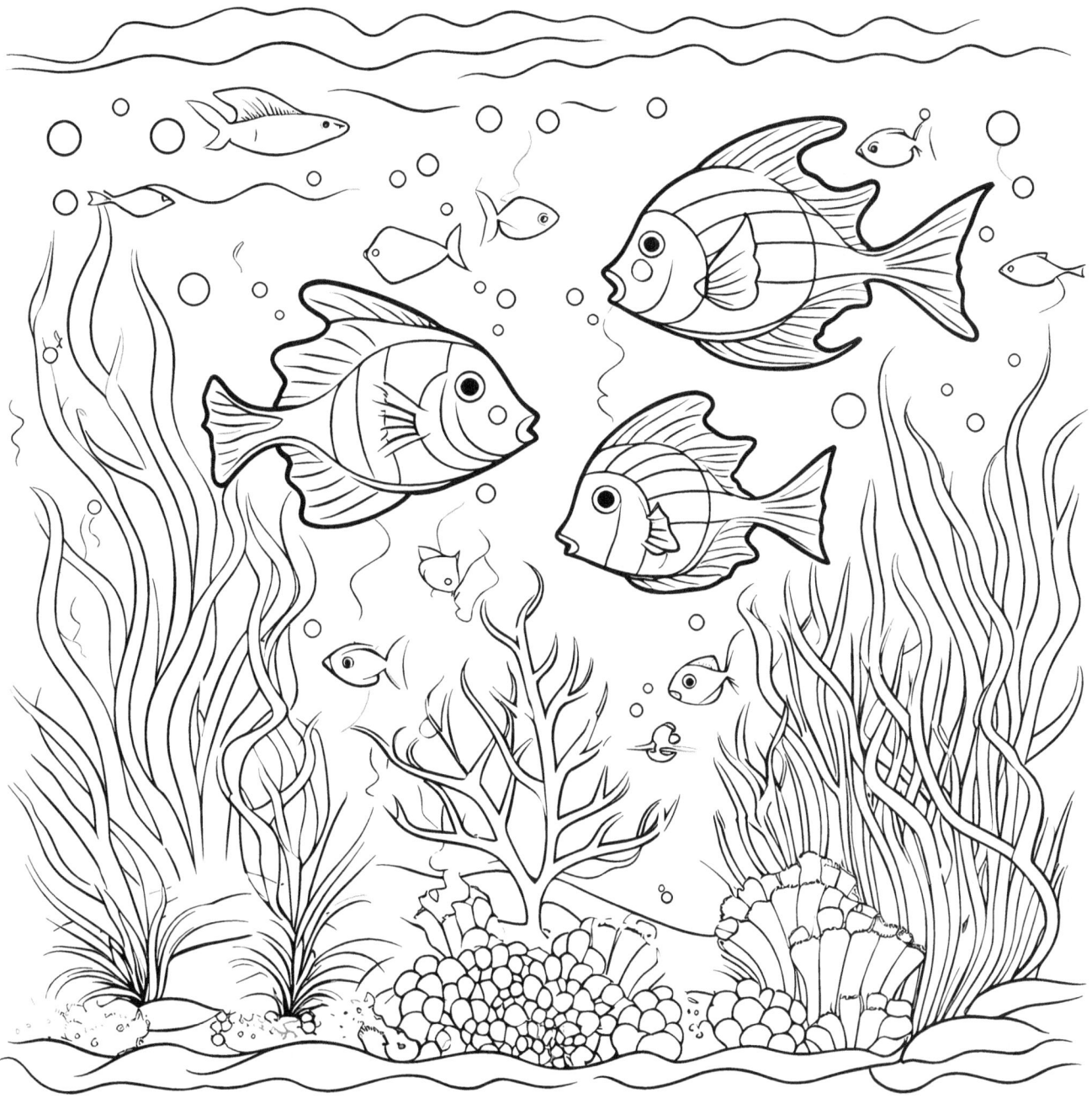

Joe Aguilus

*Blank by
Design*

Balanced Mind Balanced Life

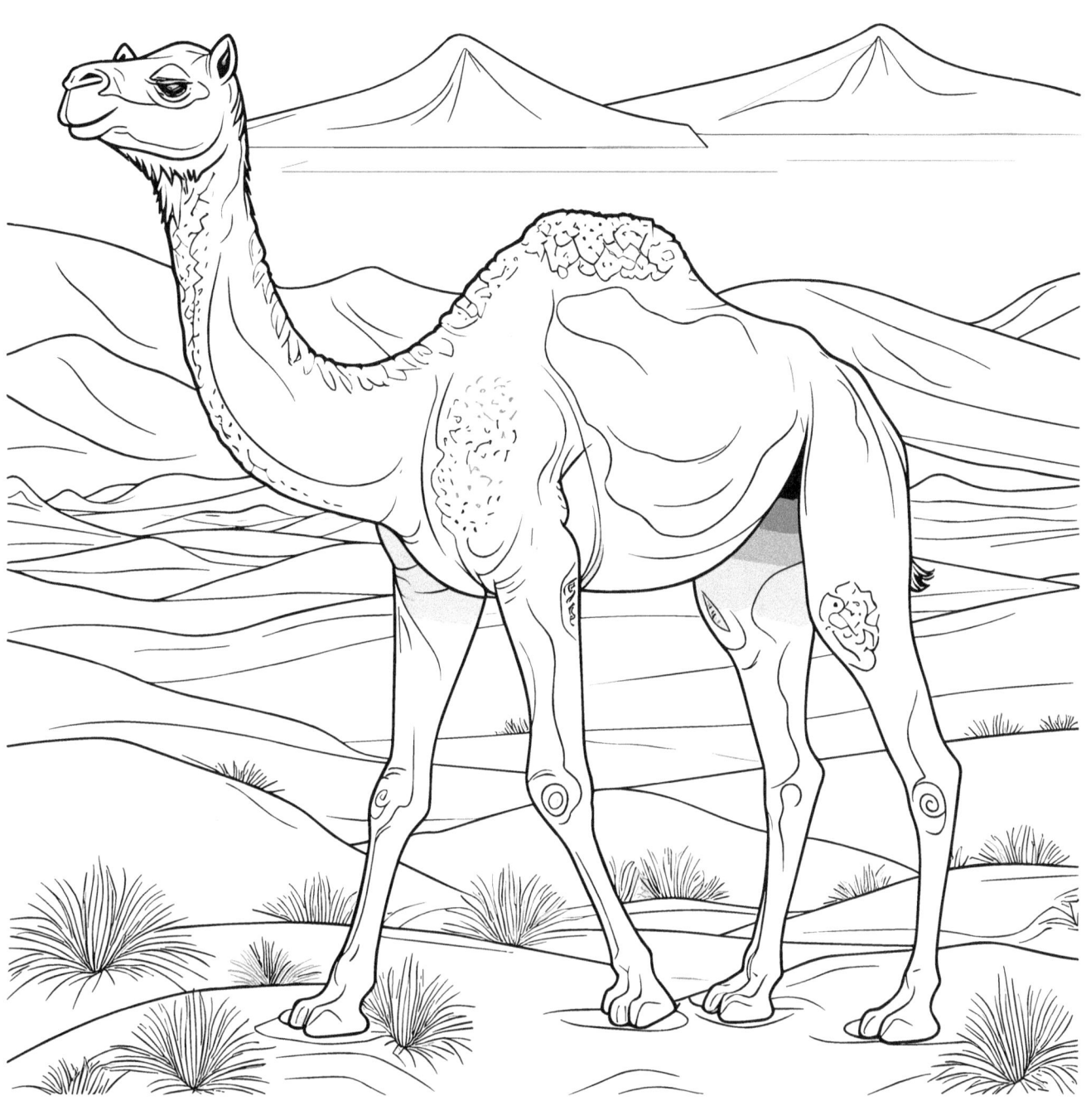

Blank by Design

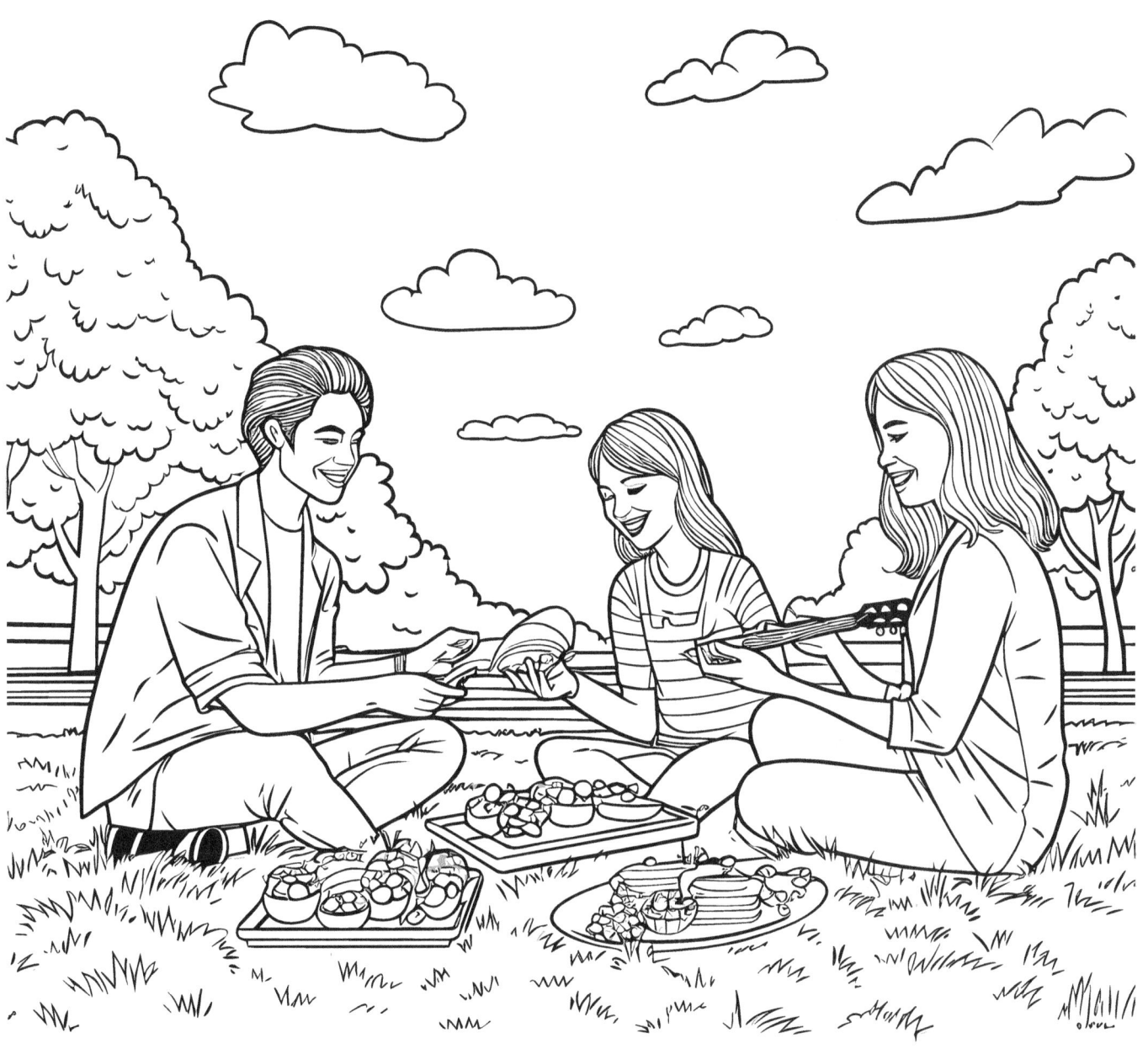

Blank by Design

Balanced Mind Balanced Life

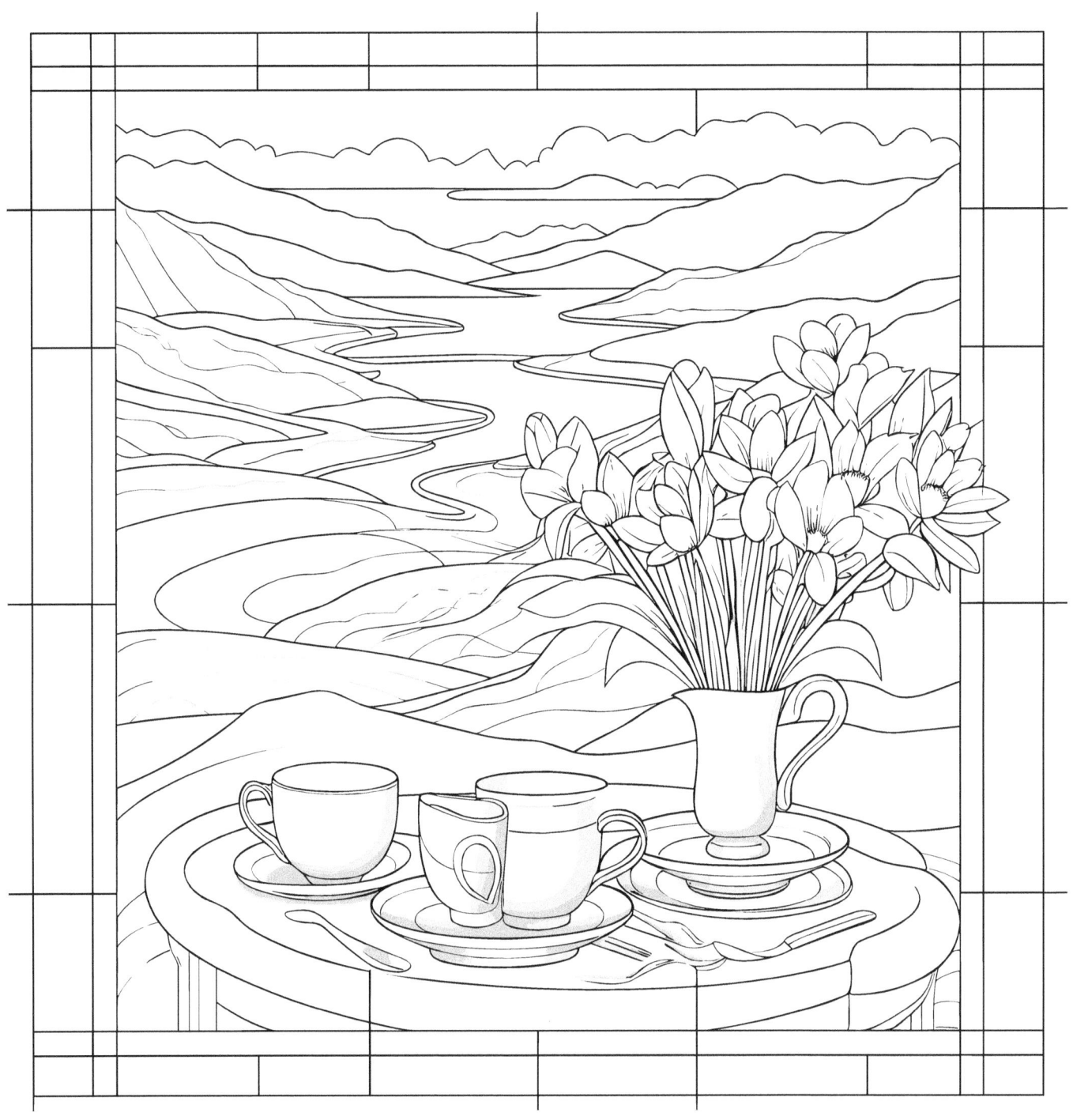

Joe Aguilus

Blank by Design

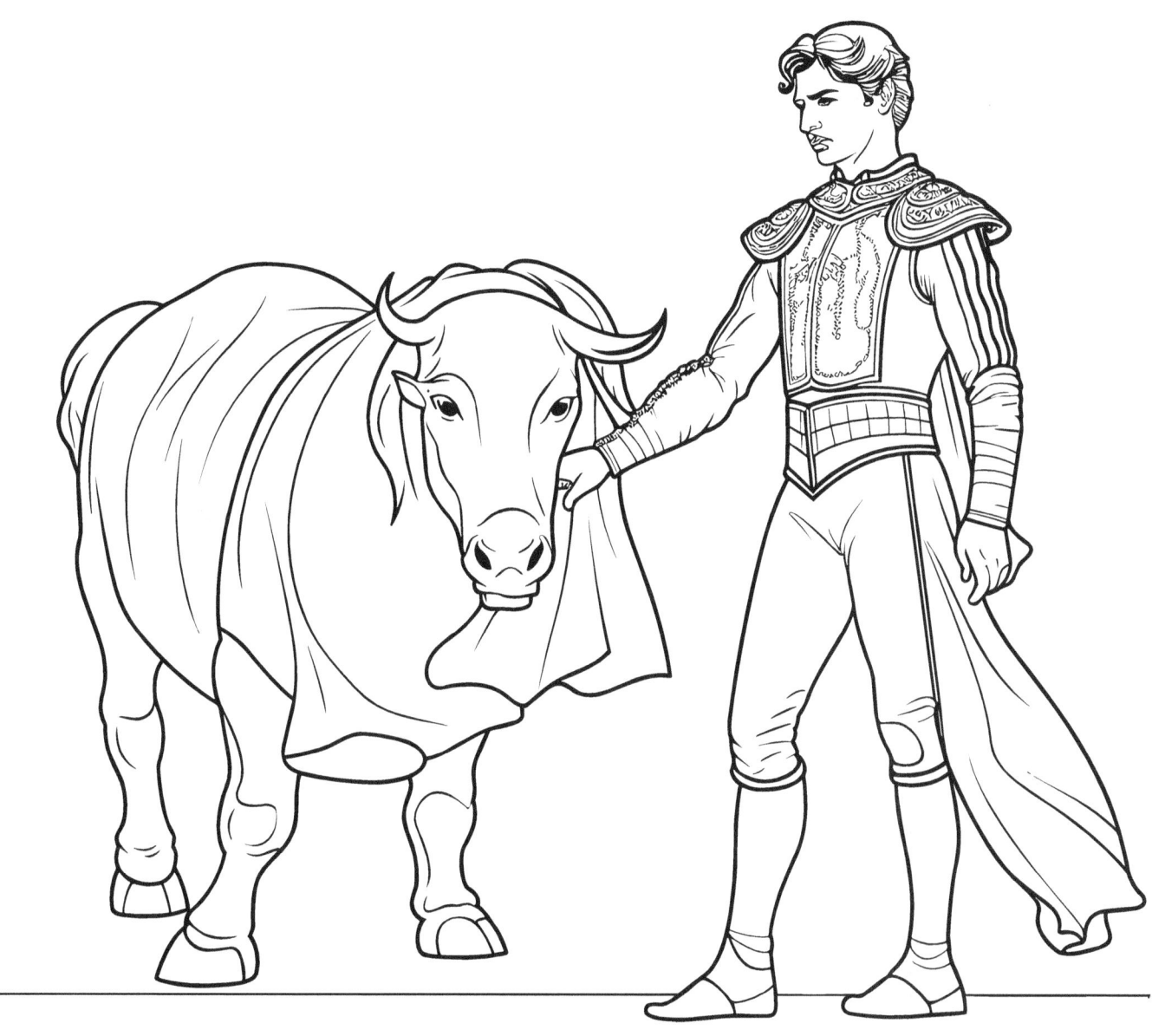

Blank by Design

Balanced Mind Balanced Life

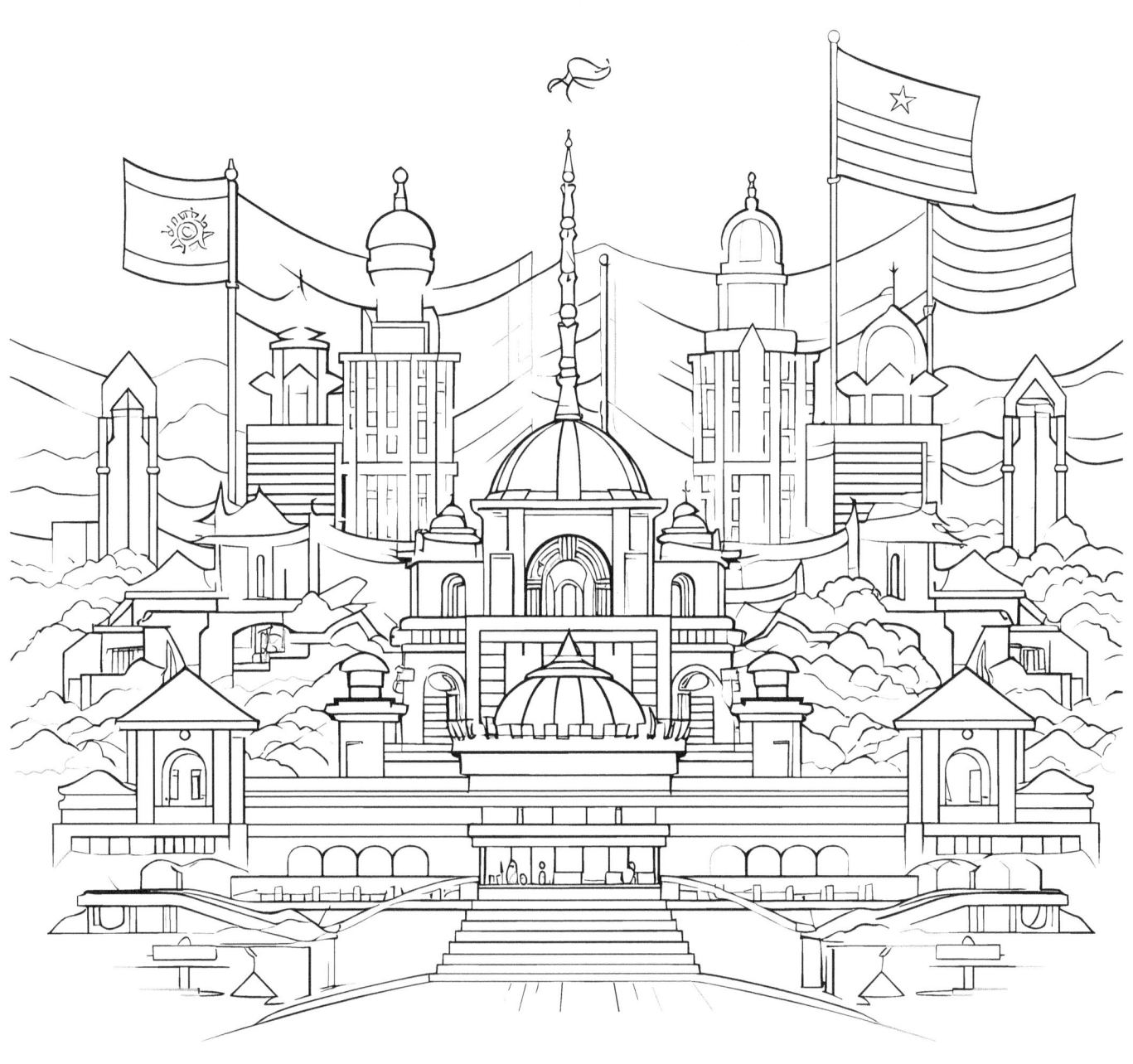

Blank by Design

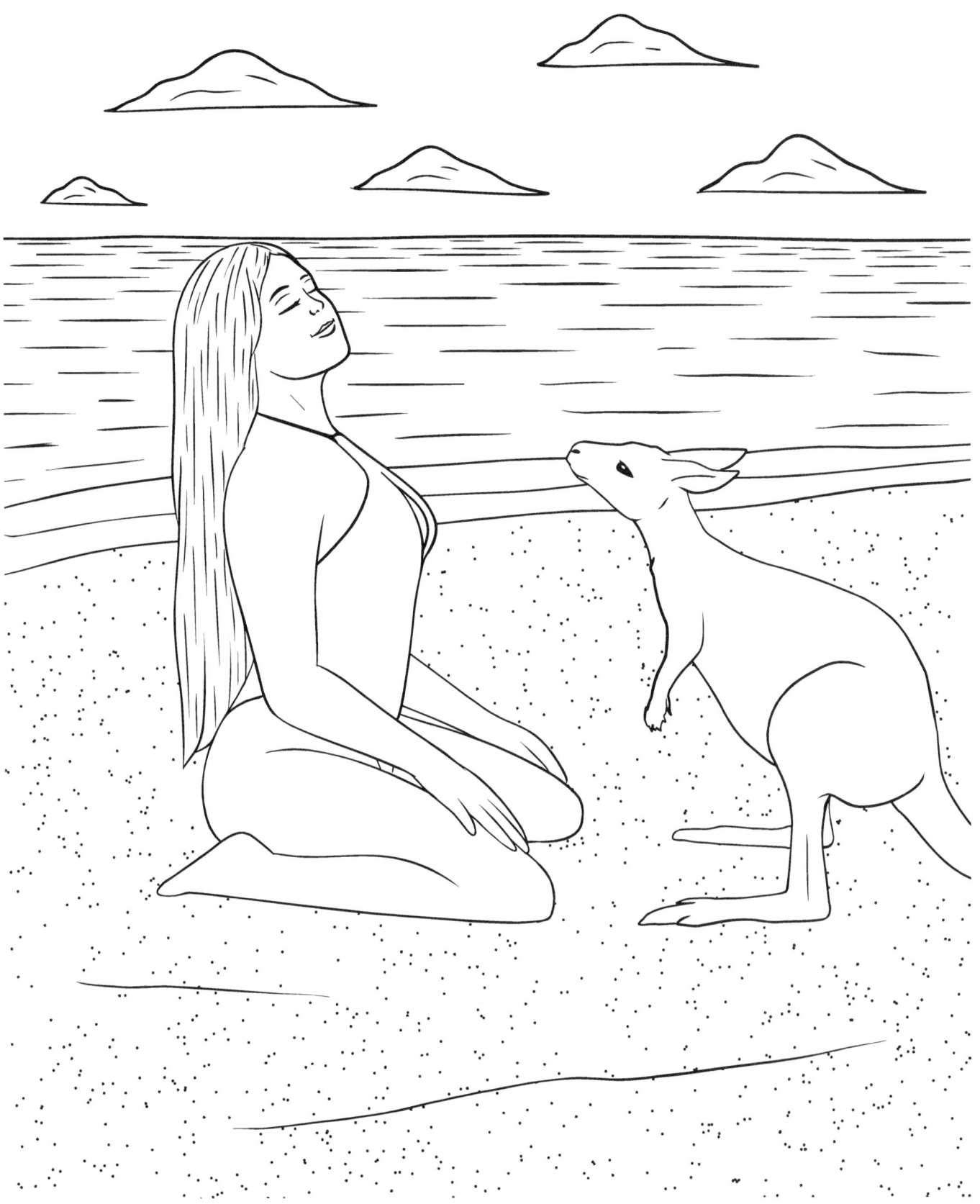

Blank by Design

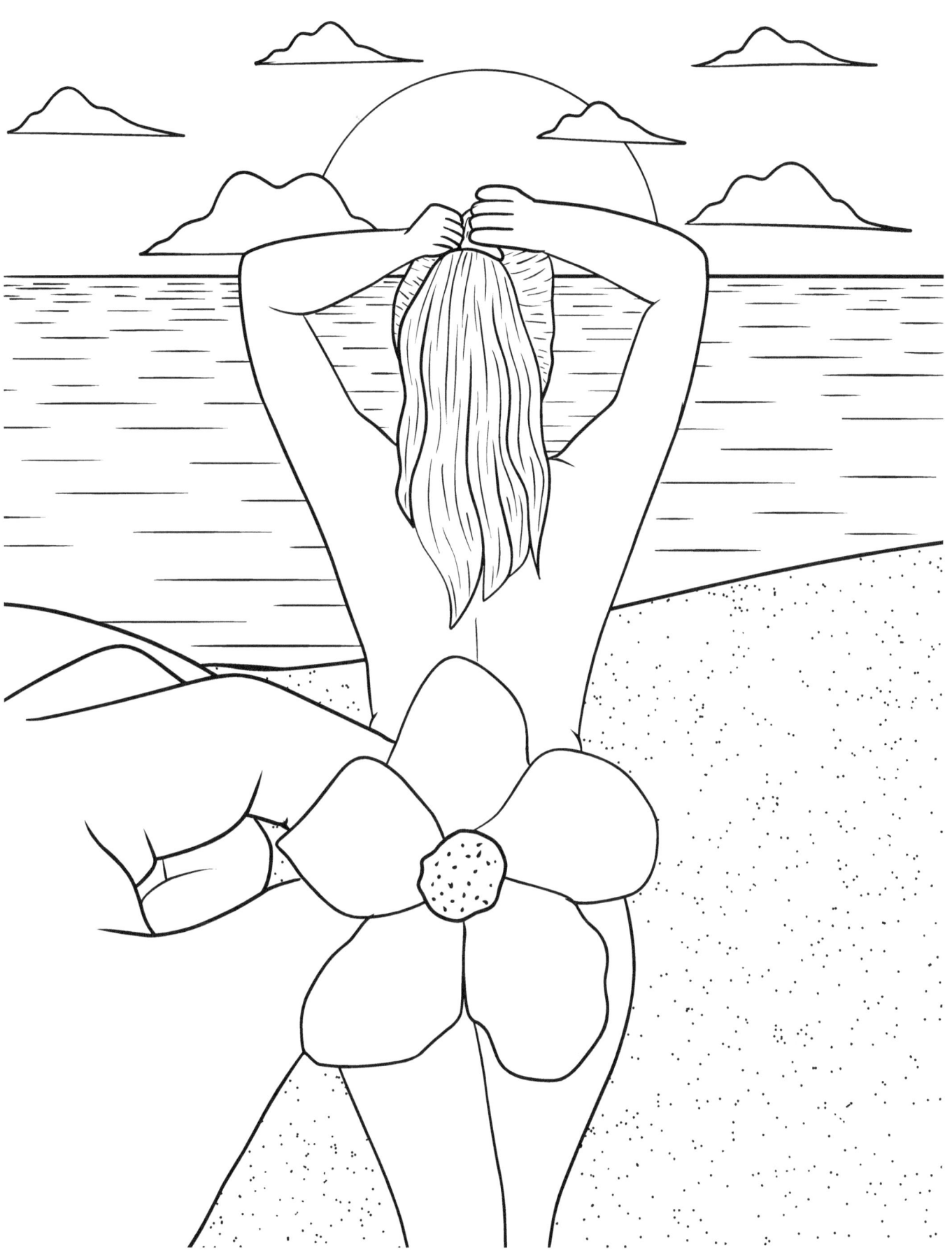

Joe Aguilus

Blank by Design

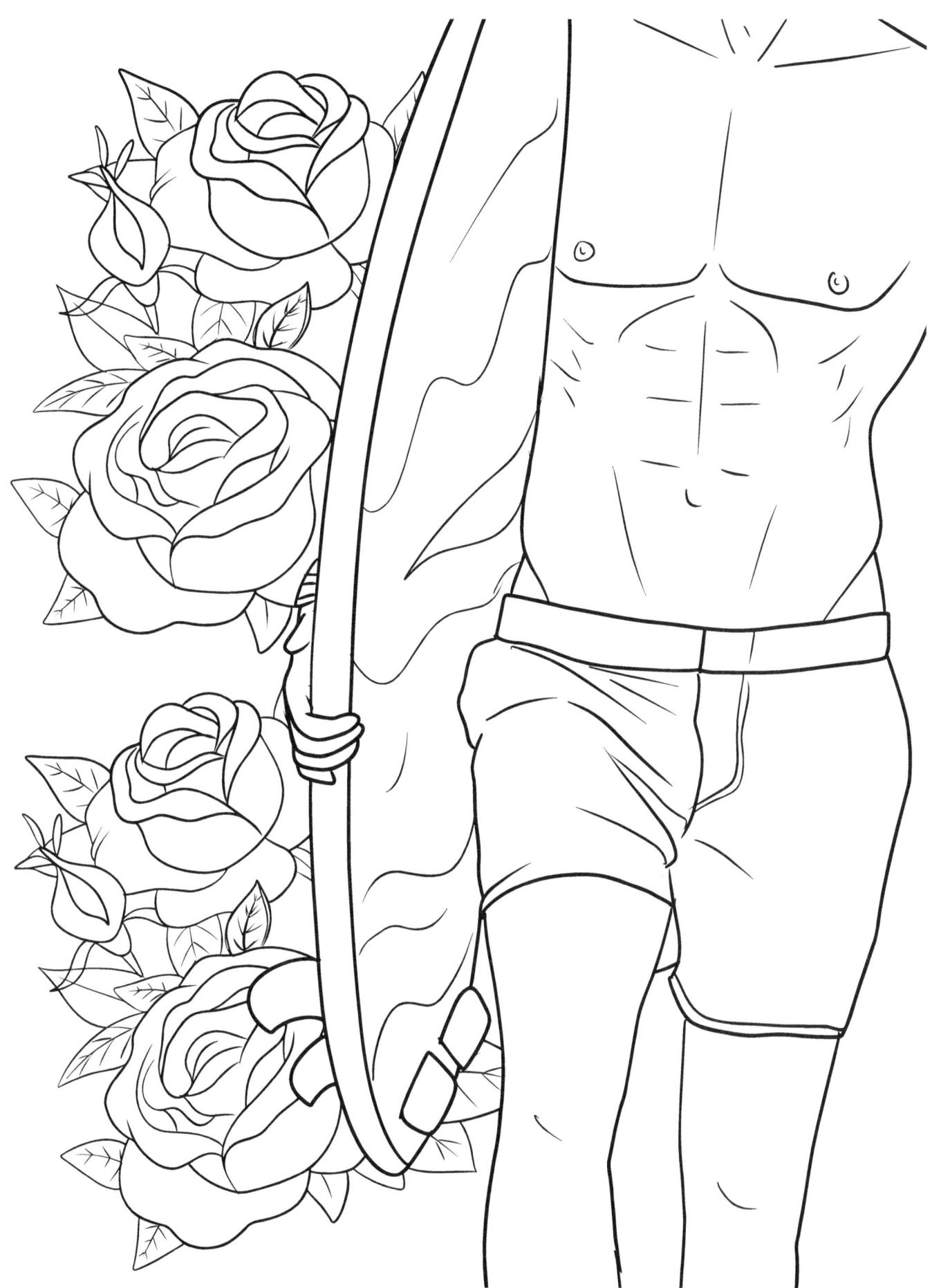

Joe Aguilus

Blank by Design

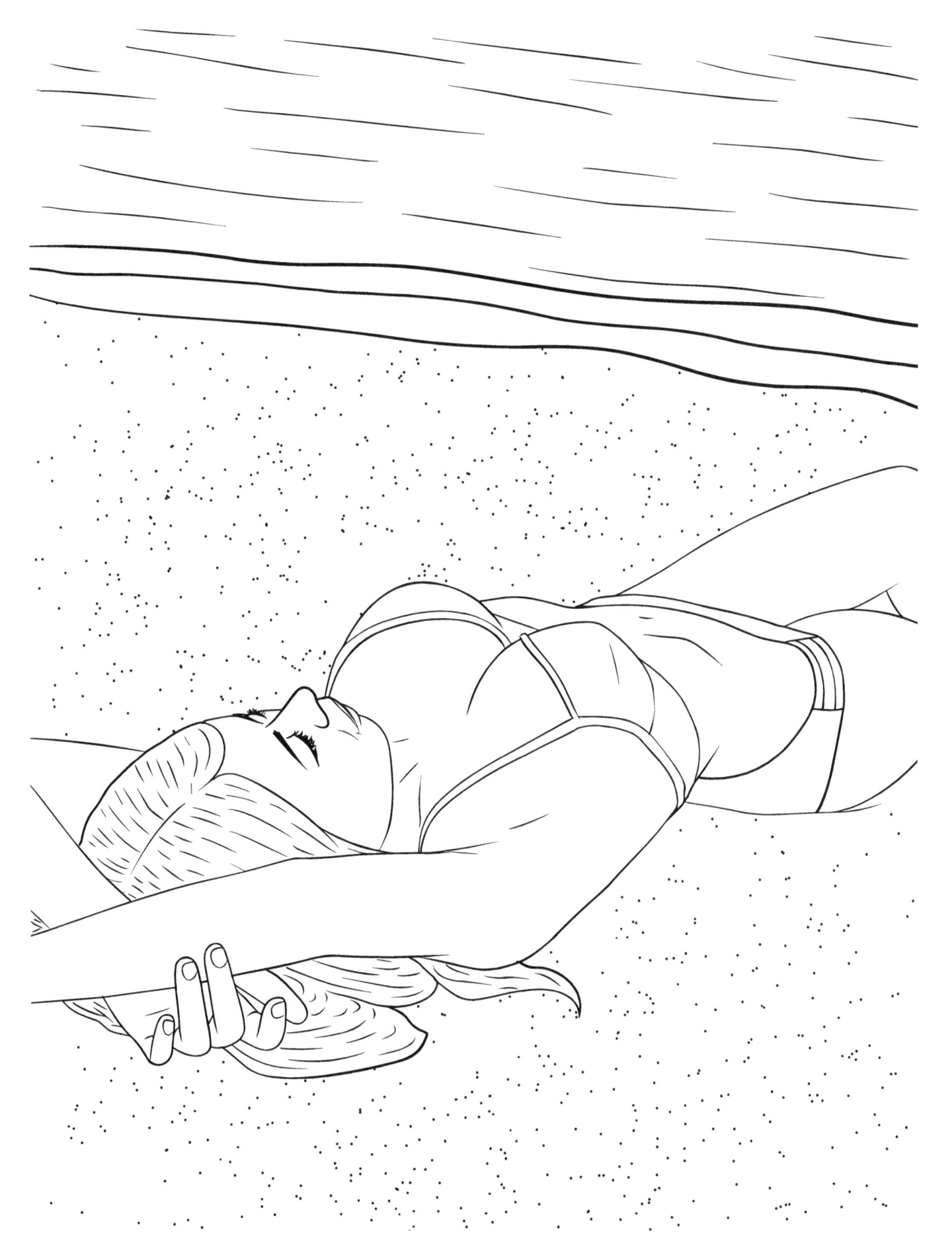

Joe Aguilus

Blank by Design

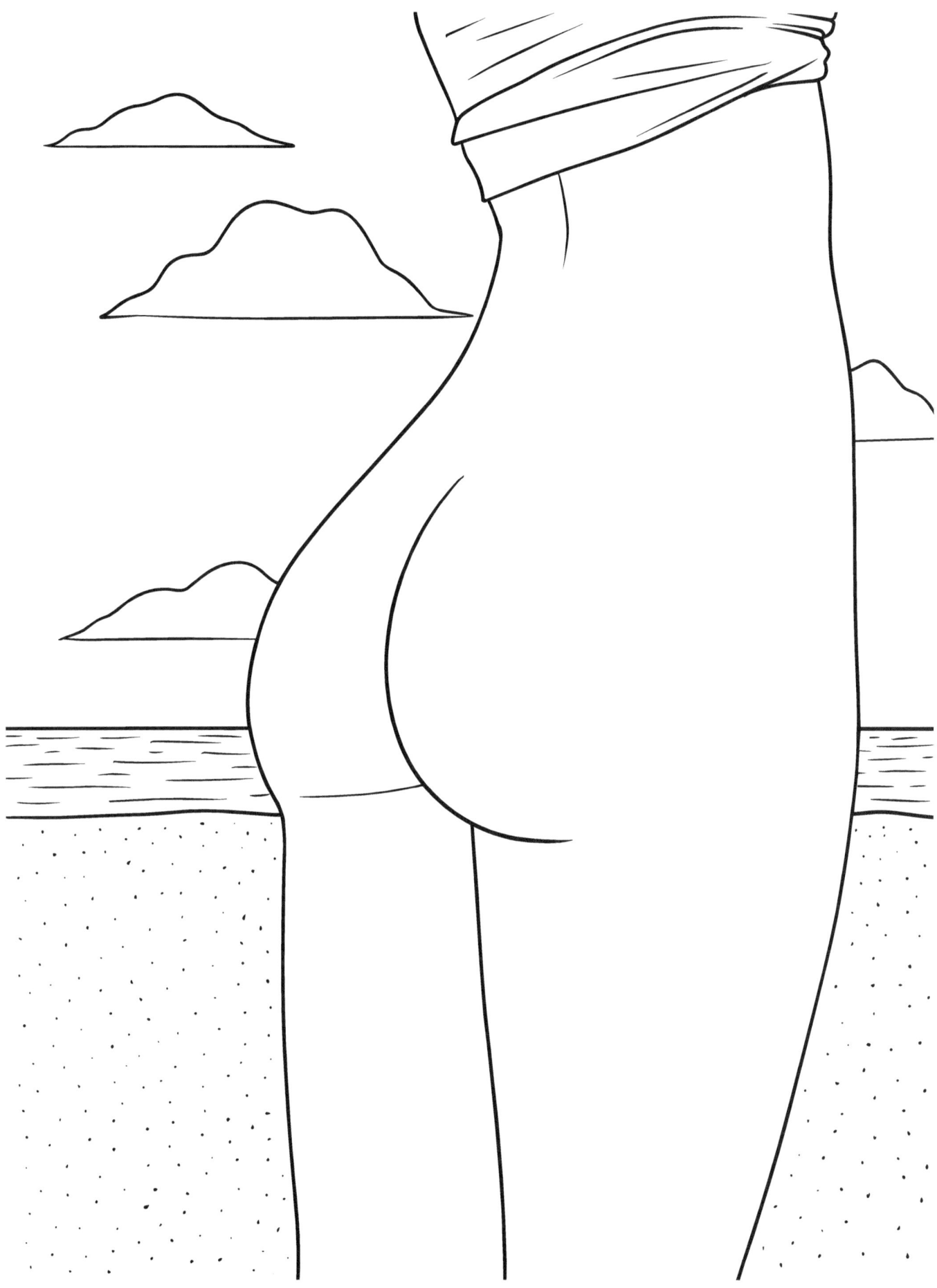

Joe Aguilus

Blank by Design

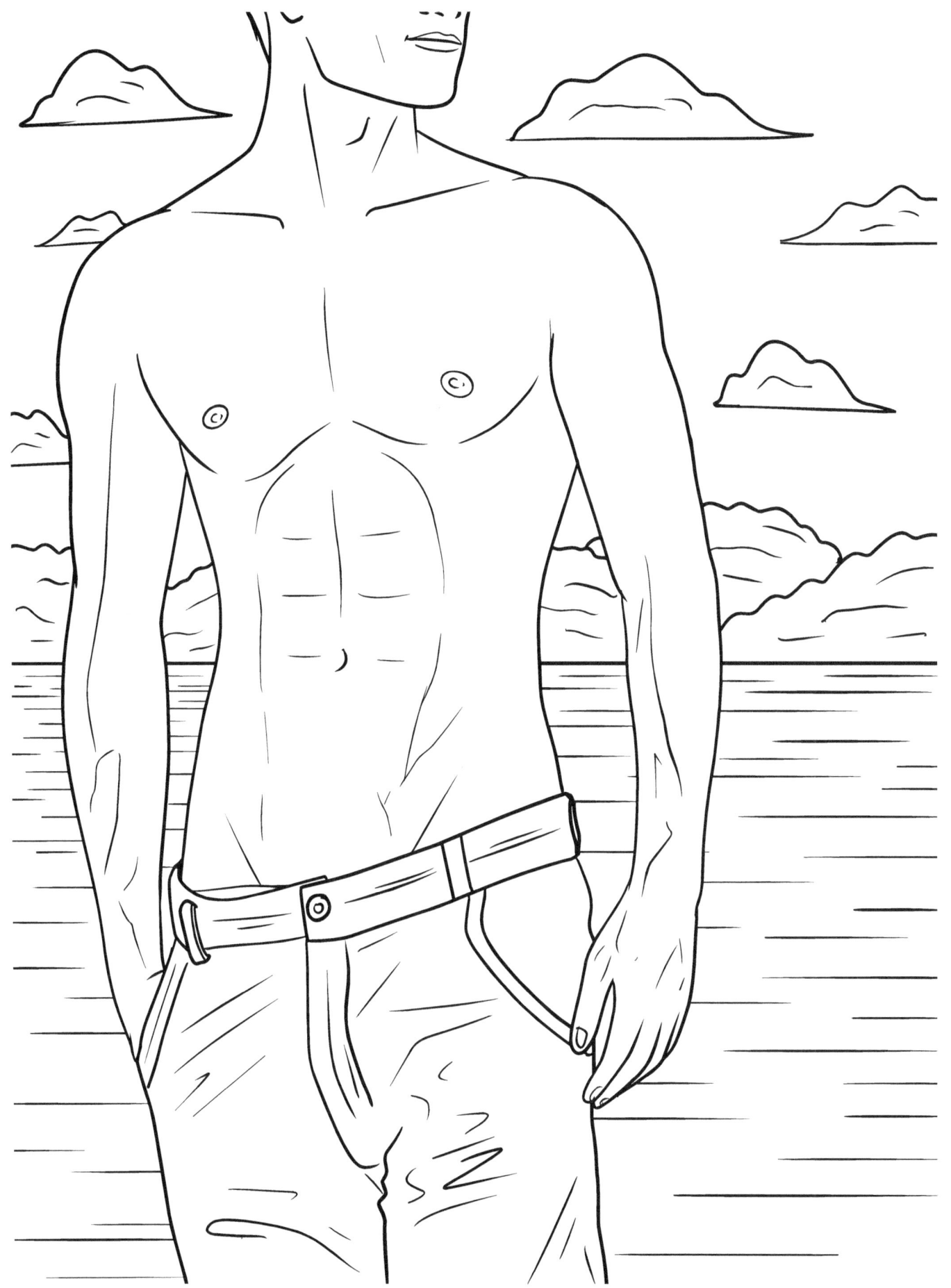

Joe Aguilus

Blank by Design

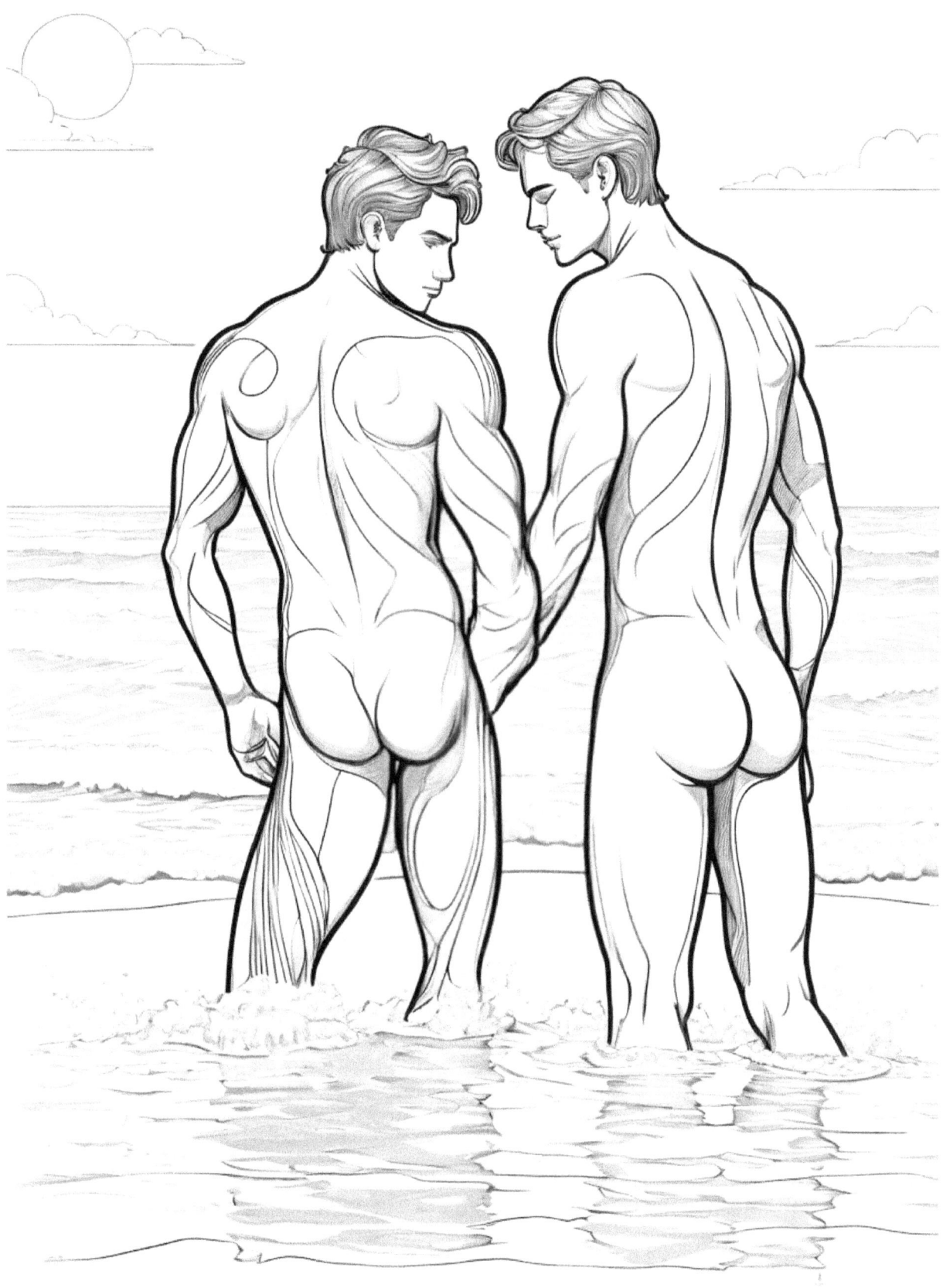

Blank by Design

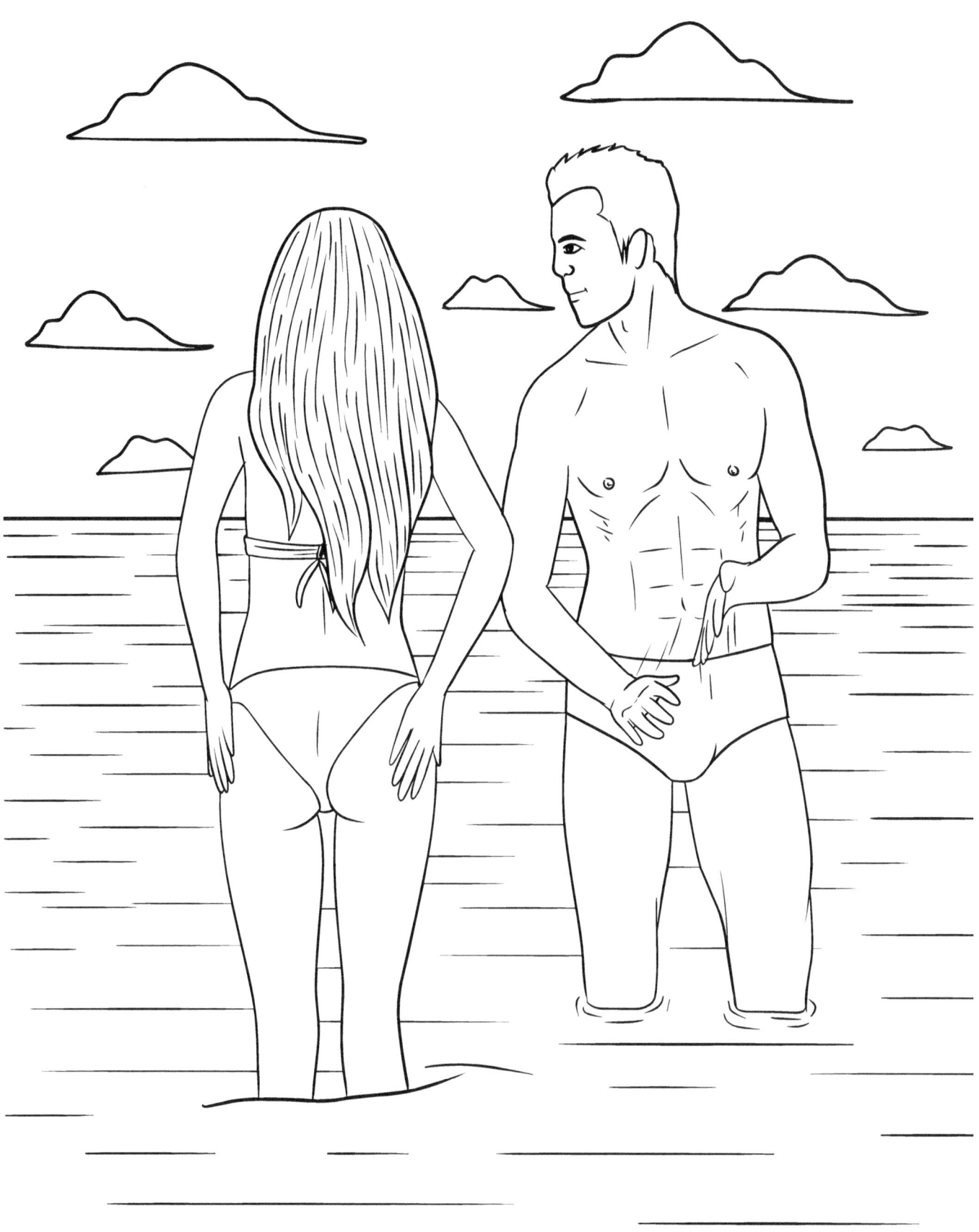

Blank by Design

🌱 Comprehensive Daily Wellness & Growth Template

A holistic guide to support your mental health and personal growth journey

How to Use This Template:

- Use it daily or adapt it to your schedule
- Fill it out either in the morning, evening, or both
- Customize sections based on your needs

Morning Practice

Daily Affirmations

1. I am worthy of love, respect, and happiness
2. I choose to embrace today's opportunities for growth
3. My challenges help me become stronger and wiser
4. I trust in my ability to handle whatever comes my way
5. My feelings are valid, and I honour them with compassion
6. I am constantly growing and evolving
7. I celebrate my progress, no matter how small

Today's Intentions

- My main focus today is: _____
- I will be gentle with myself by: _____
- I choose to let go of: _____
- I will make time for: _____

Mindfulness Practice

Choose your mindfulness activity:

- Guided meditation
- Deep breathing exercises
- Body scan meditation
- Walking meditation
- Mindful eating
- Other: _____

Duration: _____ minutes _____

Daily Action Steps

Mental Well-being

- Practice mindfulness/meditation (10 mins)
- Read something inspiring
- Take regular breaks between tasks
- Connect with a friend or loved one
- Practice positive self-talk

Physical Care

- Drink 8 glasses of water
- Move my body for 30 minutes
- Get adequate sleep (7-8 hours)
- Eat nourishing meals
- Take brief walking breaks

Personal Development

- Work on a skill for 25 minutes
- Learn something new
- Read industry/field-related content
- Network or collaborate with others
- Review and update personal goals

Creative Expression

Choose your creative outlet(s):

- Writing/Journaling
  Style: (poetry, story, free writing) _____
  - Topic/prompt: _____
- Visual Arts
  Medium: (sketching, painting, digital art) _____
  - Project: _____
- Music/Sound
  Activity: (playing instrument, singing, composing) _____
  - Piece/song: _____
- Movement/Dance

Style: _____
    ◦ Music/inspiration: _____
- Crafts/Making
  Project: (knitting, pottery, DIY) _____
    ◦ Materials needed: _____
- Photography
- Subject/theme: _____
    ◦ Location: _____

Time dedicated to creative practice: _____ minutes _____

Evening Reflection

Gratitude Practice

Today I'm grateful for:

1. _____
2. _____
3. _____

Growth Reflection

- What challenged me today? _____
- How did I handle it? _____
- What did I learn? _____
- How can I improve tomorrow? _____

Achievements

- My wins today (big or small): _____
- Progress I made toward my goals: _____
- Kind things I did for myself or others: _____
- Today, I felt most at peace when: _____
- One thing I learned about myself today: _____

Creative Practice Reflection

- How did this creative activity make me feel? _____
- What did I discover or learn? _____
- Ideas for tomorrow's creative practice: _____

Tomorrow's Preparation

- Top 3 priorities for tomorrow:
  1. _____
  2. _____
  3. _____

- One thing I'm looking forward to: _____
- Self-care activity I'll prioritize: _____

Weekly Review Section (Complete on Sundays)

Progress Review

- Skills I developed: _____
- Habits I maintained: _____
- Challenges I overcame: _____
- Areas for improvement: _____
- Positive changes in my mental health/mindset: _____
- Most impactful daily actions: _____
- Recurring thoughts or challenges to address: _____

Goal Setting

- Next week's focus area: _____
- One new habit to implement: _____
- One limiting belief to work on: _____
- One act of self-care to prioritize: _____
- My intention for next week: _____

Remember: Progress isn't linear. Every step forward counts, no matter how small. Be patient and kind with yourself as you grow. 🌱

Bibliography:

'Aurelius, Marcus', *Marcus Aurelius Quotes* (Web Page) <https://www.brainyquote.com/quotes/marcus_aurelius_131341>

'Australian Institute of Health and Welfare', *Prevalence and impact of mental illness* (Web Page) < https://www.aihw.gov.au/mental-health/overview/prevalence-and-impact-of-mental-illness>

'BBC Food', *How diet can affect your mental wellbeing* (Web Page) <https://www.bbc.co.uk/food/articles/diet_wellbeing>

Brown-Grant, K, GW Harris and S Reichlin, 'The effect of emotional and physical stress on thyroid activity in the rabbit' (1954) 126(1) *The Journal of Physiology* 29

Carcedo, Rodrigo J et al, 'Association between sexual satisfaction and depression and anxiety in adolescents and young adults' (2020) 17(3) *International journal of environmental research and public health* 1

'Cherry, Kendra', *How you can strengthen your brain with exercises* (Web Page) <https://www.verywellmind.com/brain-exercises-to-strengthen-your-mind-2795039>

'Dekker, Thomas', *Thomas Dekker Quotes* (Web Page) <https://www.goodreads.com/author/quotes/22587.Thomas_Dekker>

'Dementia Australia', *How do our brains work?* (Web Page) <https://www.dementia.org.au/news/how-do-our-brains-work>

'Edison, Thomas A', *Thomas A. Edison Quotes* (Web Page) <https://www.brainyquote.com/quotes/thomas_a_edison_1063850>

Eichenseher, Tasha, 'How to develop self-awareness and why it's important' (Media Release, 21 April 2022) <https://psychcentral.com/health/self-awareness>

Engel, George L., 'The Clinical Application of the Biopsychosocial Model' (1981) 6(2) *The Journal of Medicine and Philosophy: A Forum for Bioethics and Philosophy of Medicine* 101

'Gandhi, Mahatma', *Mahatma Gandhi Quotes* (Web Page) <https://www.brainyquote.com/quotes/mahatma_gandhi_109078>

'Good Housekeeping', *45 inspirational mental health quotes* (Web Page) <https://www.goodhousekeeping.com/life/a39739060/mental-health-quotes/>

'Gunnars, Kris', *How to overcome food addiction* (Web Page) <https://www.healthline.com/nutrition/how-to-overcome-food-addiction>

'Hamblen, Jessica', *What is PTSD? A handout from the National Center for PTSD* (Web Page) <http://www.ncptsd.va.gov/ncmain/ncdocs/handouts/handout_What%20is%20PTSD.pdf>

Heger, Erin and John Mutziger, '4 reasons why self-awareness matters and 3 ways to develop it' (Media Release, 20 January 2022) <https://www.businessinsider.nl/4-reasons-why-self-awareness-matters-and-3-ways-to-develop-it/>

'Holland, Kimberly', *How many cups of coffee a day are safe?* (Web Page) <https://www.healthline.com/health-news/6-cups-of-coffee-a-day-is-safe-but-more-isnt-healthy>

'Humphries, Barry', *50+ Ripper Australian quotes, slang and sayings* (Web Page) <https://aussietourist.com.au/australian-quotes-instagram-captions/>

'Jacka, Felice', *The fascinating connection between diet and depression* (Web Page) <https://this.deakin.edu.au/self-improvement/the-fascinating-connection-between-diet-and-depression>

Jacka, Felice N et al, 'A randomised controlled trial of dietary improvement for adults with major depression (the 'SMILES' trial)' (2017) 15(1) *BMC Medicine* 1

'Johns Hopkins Medicine', *Mental Health Disorder Statistics* (web Page) <https://www.hopkinsmedicine.org/health/wellness-and-prevention/mental-health-disorder-statistics>

'Matejko, Sonya', *What's the background of mindfulness?* (Web Page) <https://psychcentral.com/lib/a-brief-history-of-mindfulness-in-the-usa-and-its-impact-on-our-lives>

'Mental Health Foundation', *Diet and mental health* (Web Page) <https://www.mentalhealth.org.uk/explore-mental-health/a-z-topics/diet-and-mental-health>

'Mental Health Foundation', *How to look after your mental health using exercise* (Web Page) <https://www.mentalhealth.org.uk/explore-mental-health/publications/how-look-after-your-mental-health-using-exercise>

'Medical News Today', *Vitamin D: Benefits, deficiency, sources, and dosage* (Web Page) <https://www.medicalnewstoday.com/articles/161618>

'Mind', *Mindfulness* (Web Page) <https://www.mind.org.uk/information-support/drugs-and-treatments/mindfulness/about-mindfulness/>

'Mindmaps.com', *What is mind mapping? What are its uses?* (Web Page) <https://www.mindmaps.com/what-is-mind-mapping/>

Mizokami, Tetsuya et al, 'Stress and Thyroid Autoimmunity' (2004) 14(12) *Thyroid* 1047

Molendijk, Marc et al, 'Diet quality and depression risk: A systematic review and dose-response meta-analysis of prospective studies' (2018) 226 *Journal of Affective Disorders* 346

'National Institute of General Medical Sciences', *Circadian Rhythms* (Web Page) <https://bilimblogum.wordpress.com/wp-content/uploads/2022/11/fact-sheet-circadian-rhythms.pdf>

Nikolin, Steven et al, 'An investigation of working memory deficits in depression using the n-back task: A systematic review and meta-analysis' (2021) 284 *Journal of Affective Disorders* 1

'Newsom, Rob', *Blue Light: what it is and how it affects sleep* (Web Page) <https://www.sleepfoundation.org/bedroom-environment/blue-light>

Perrotta, Giulio, 'Psychological Trauma: Definition, Clinical Contexts, Neural Correlates and Therapeutic Approaches Recent Discoveries' [2019] (1) *Current Research in Psychiatry and Brain Disorders* 1

Petra, Anastasia I et al, 'Gut-microbiota-brain axis and its effect on neuropsychiatric disorders with suspected immune dysregulation' (2022) 44(1) *Clinical Therapeutics* 10

Sarris, Jerome et al, 'Nutritional psychiatry: the present state of the evidence' (2020) 76(4) *Proceedings of the Nutrition Society* 427

Sathyanarayana Rao, T S et al, 'Understanding nutrition, depression and mental illnesses' (2008) 50(2) *Indian Journal of Psychiatry* 77

Schneiderman, Neil, Gail Ironson, and Scott D. Siege, 'Stress and health: Psychological, behavioural, and biological determinants' (2005) 1(1) *Annual Review of Clinical Psychology* 607

'Scott, Jess C', *Jess C Scott Quotes* (Web Page) <https://www.wisdomtimes.com/quotes/author/jess-c-scott/>

'Sima, Richard', *The mental health benefits of reading* (Web Page) <https://www.psychologytoday.com/us/blog/the-art-effect/202203/the-mental-health-benefits-reading>

'Stevenson, Robert Louis', *Robert Louis Stevenson Quotes* (Web Page) <https://www.brainyquote.com/quotes/robert_louis_stevenson_101230>

'Suni, Eric', *Mental Health and Sleep* (Web Page) <https://www.sleepfoundation.org/mental-health>

'United Nations', *Nearly one billion people have a mental disorder: WHO* (Web Page) <https://news.un.org/en/story/2022/06/1120682>

Wahl, Siegfried et al, 'The inner clock – Blue light sets the human rhythm' (2019) 12(12) *Journal of Biophotonics* 1

'World Health Organization', *Mental disorders* (Web Page) <https://www.who.int/news-room/fact-sheets/detail/mental-disorders>

Useful Resources

If you're facing anxiety and depression, there are various ways to seek support:

Professional Help in Australia

General Practitioners (GPs)

Your GP is often the ideal first step. They can:

- Assess your mental health
- Provide initial treatment
- Refer you to mental health specialists as needed
- Develop a mental health treatment plan for Medicare rebates

Mental Health Specialists

- **Psychologists:** They diagnose and treat mental health issues using therapies like cognitive behavioural therapy (CBT) and mindfulness-based cognitive therapy.
- **Psychiatrists:** These medical doctors specialize in mental health, capable of prescribing medication and offering psychotherapy.
- **Counsellors and Psychotherapists:** They assist those dealing with mental health challenges, relationships, grief, or addiction.

Helplines and Online Support

- **Beyond Blue:** Call 1300 22 4636 (available 24/7) or use their online chat service.
- **Lifeline:** Contact 13 11 14 (available 24/7) for crisis support and suicide prevention.
- **Headspace:** Provides free online and phone counselling for individuals aged 12-25.

Online Resources and Programs

- **MindSpot Clinic:** Offers free online and telephone treatment for anxiety and depression.
- **This Way Up:** Provides an internet-based treatment program for anxiety and depression.
- **Black Dog Institute:** Offers information about mental health issues and self-tests.
- **Head to Health:** A government website that connects you to mental health services and information.

Support Groups

Many communities host support groups for those experiencing anxiety and depression, providing a safe space to share experiences and learn from others.

Finding the Right Professional

Finding a professional you feel comfortable with is crucial. While some may find the right fit on their first try, others might need to explore a bit longer. Don't be discouraged by a negative experience; seeking help is a sign of strength, not weakness. If you're feeling overwhelmed, reach out to these services or a trusted person in your life.

Remember, everyone's journey is unique, and it may take time to discover the support that works best for you.

www.ingramcontent.com/pod-product-compliance
Lightning Source LLC
Chambersburg PA
CBHW060419300426
44111CB00018B/2901